Goal Setting in Speech-Language Pathology

A GUIDE TO CLINICAL REASONING

T0371878

Goal Setting in Speech-Language Pathology

A GUIDE TO CLINICAL REASONING

Casey Taliancich-Klinger, PhD, CCC-SLP
Angela J. Kennedy, SLPD, CCC-SLP
Catherine Torrington Eaton, PhD, CCC-SLP

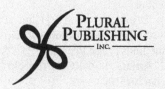

PLURAL
PUBLISHING
INC.

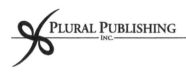

9177 Aero Drive, Suite B
San Diego, CA 92123

email: information@pluralpublishing.com
website: https://www.pluralpublishing.com

Typeset in 12.5/15 Minion Pro by Achorn International, Inc.
Printed in the United States of America by Integrated Books International

Library of Congress Cataloging-in-Publication Data:
Names: Taliancich-Klinger, Casey, author. | Kennedy, Angela J., author. |
    Eaton, Catherine Torrington, author.
Title: Goal setting in speech-language pathology : a guide to clinical reasoning /
    Casey Taliancich-Klinger, Angela J. Kennedy, Catherine Torrington Eaton.
Description: San Diego, CA : Plural Publishing, [2025] | Includes bibliographical
    references and index.
Identifiers: LCCN 2023030318 (print) | LCCN 2023030319 (ebook) |
    ISBN 9781635504323 (paperback) | ISBN 1635504325 (paperback) |
    ISBN 9781635504330 (ebook)
Subjects: MESH: Language Disorders—therapy | Clinical Reasoning | Child |
    Patient Care Planning—standards | Professional-Patient Relations | Speech-
    Language Pathology—methods | Case Reports
Classification: LCC RC427 (print) | LCC RC427 (ebook) | NLM WL 340.2 |
    DDC 616.85/5—dc23/eng/20231003
LC record available at https://lccn.loc.gov/2023030318
LC ebook record available at https://lccn.loc.gov/2023030319

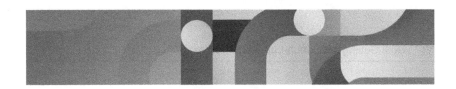

Contents

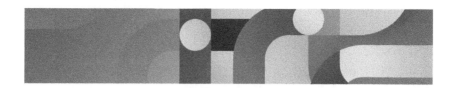

Introduction

Are you struggling with how to move from diagnostic information to patient-centered, functional goals? If so, this is
the resource for you!

We encourage you to start at the beginning so that we share
a common terminology and cognitive framework. You will then
be equipped to engage with the case studies that allow you to
practice clinical reasoning across a variety of disorders, patient
ages, and settings. You can use this resource independently
to develop or enhance your clinical reasoning skills or work
through it with an instructor or clinical supervisor for the additional benefit of their expert knowledge.

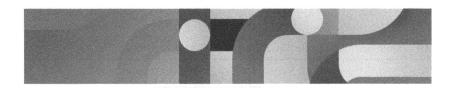

About the Authors

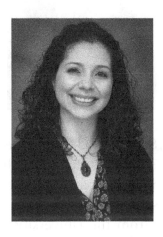

Casey Taliancich-Klinger, PhD, CCC-SLP, is a bilingual speech-language pathologist, researcher, and Project Director. She holds a PhD in speech-language pathology from the University of Texas at Austin, where she also earned her MA in speech-language pathology, BA in Spanish, and BA in communication sciences and disorders. Dr. Taliancich-Klinger currently serves as an adjunct Assistant Professor in the Department of Communication Sciences and Disorders at UT Health San Antonio, and as a project director for Western Psychological Services. Her research focuses on language characteristics of Spanish-English bilingual children, multicultural issues, and graduate student learning. Together with a non-profit partner, Dr. Taliancich-Klinger codirects a community engagement pediatric clinical experience for graduate students and is passionate about fostering inter-professional collaborations within the field of speech-language pathology and other health professions.

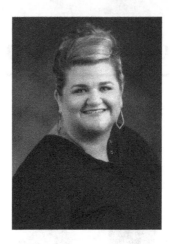

Angela J. Kennedy, SLPD, CCC-SLP, is the Director of Clinical Education and an Assistant Professor for the Speech-Language Pathology program in the Department of Communication Sciences and Disorders. She received her BA and MA in speech-language pathology from the University of North Texas and completed her clinical doctorate in speech-language pathology from Northwestern University. She has over 15 years of clinical experience in pediatric speech-language pathology in a variety of clinical settings including school-based, pediatric outpatient, home health, and university-based settings. Her current areas of research interest include increasing access to rehabilitative services for pediatric patients with communication disorders in under-resourced areas, examining the training and equipping of speech-language pathologists specifically in the area of speech sound disorders, and the implementation of interprofessional clinically based activities in graduate-level curriculums.

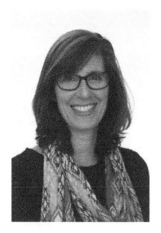

Catherine Torrington Eaton, PhD, CCC-SLP, is an Assistant Professor in the Department of Communication Sciences and Disorders at the University of Texas Health Science Center in San Antonio, Texas. She has worked as a speech-language patholo-gist in various medical and education settings, but her clinical specialty is aphasia. Her primary research interests include func-tional language use in patients with post-stroke and primary progressive aphasia as well as communication partner training for healthcare providers. Dr. Eaton teaches graduate courses in neuroanatomy and neurophysiology, clinical methods, and neurogenic language disorders, and she loves the challenge of clinical supervision.

Acknowledgments

Thank you to fellow clinicians who gave us advice on the content: April Duvall, Rey Piña, and others. We are grateful to our patients whose stories informed this work and inspired us to do better. Finally, we would like to thank the University of Texas Health San Antonio graduate class of 2024 for being our guinea pigs in piloting this framework and—in general—knocking it out of the park.

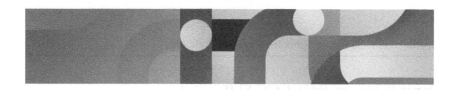

Reviewers

Plural Publishing and the authors would like to thank the following reviewers for taking the time to provide their valuable feedback during the manuscript development process. Additional anonymous feedback was provided by other expert reviewers.

Adrienne Bratcher, SLPD, CCC-SLP, BSIST
Professor and Health & Human Services
    Department Chair
Eastern New Mexico University
Portales, New Mexico

Krista R. Davidson, MS, CCC-SLP
Clinical Associate Professor
The University of Iowa
Iowa City, Iowa

Melissa P. Garcia, EdD, CCC-SLP
Clinical Assistant Professor
Baylor University
Waco, Texas

Joy Kennedy, MEd, PhD
Assistant Professor
North Carolina Agricultural and Technical State
    University
Greensboro, North Carolina

Janie P. Magee, EdD, CCC-SLP
Clinical Director and Faculty
Delta State University
Cleveland, Mississippi

Juliana O. Miller, MS, CCC-SLP
Clinical Assistant Professor and Director of External
    Clinical Practicum
University of South Carolina
Columbia, South Carolina

Mary P. Mitchell, PhD, CCC-SLP
Assistant Professor
School of Communication Sciences and Disorders
Pacific University
Forest Grove, Oregon

David M. Rehfeld, PhD, BCBA, CCC-SLP
Assistant Professor
Donna Nigh Department of Advanced Professional
    and Special Services
University of Central Oklahoma
Edmond, Oklahoma

Lauren Siemers, MS-SLP, BS
Director of Clinical Education and Instructor
University of Central Missouri
Warrensburg, Missouri

Meagan Spencer, EdD, CCC-SLP
Program Coordinator
Freed-Hardeman University
Henderson, Tennessee

Amy Vaughn, PhD, CCC-SLP
Associate Professor
Baldwin Wallace University
Berea, Ohio

Miriam Velsor, MA, CCC-SLP
Clinical Instructor and Adjunct Faculty
Adelphi University
Garden City, New York

*To the next generation
of speech-language pathologists
who strive to make the world a better place,
one goal at a time.*

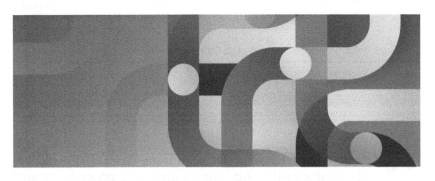

1 Clinical Reasoning Introduction

The Value-Add

We have all been there. You feel prepared from your graduate coursework. You know diagnostic procedures and have collected excellent data. Developmental norms and medical etiologies are fresh in your mind. You have administered assessments, conducted an in-depth interview with the family, and observed the client in functional interactions. The data are comprehensive and your knowledge is solid. As you have been taught, you next sit down to write three to four objective, measurable, timely, and functional goals. The problem: you are paralyzed as to where to go from here. You struggle to synthesize the information that you have gathered to write even one patient-centered goal.

Navigating the clinical decisions needed to establish functional and relevant treatment goals can feel overwhelming and even impossible. YOU ARE NOT ALONE. Feelings of frustration and inadequacy are common. After combined years of working with graduate students, we, as educators, have identified what you are experiencing: difficulty navigating the complexity of clinical reasoning in goal planning. We argue that clinical reasoning is not a skill that is innate, but a skill that must be taught and practiced in order to master.

Here are some examples taken from personal experience. Can you identify what is wrong in these scenarios?

1. A graduate clinician evaluates a 7-year-old child with minimal language skills (Mean Length of Utterance is 3.5) and severely impaired intelligibility due to speech sound substitutions. During the evaluation, she is fascinated to discover that the child cannot whisper. She proposes a goal to her clinical supervisor that the child work on whispering, which could be a helpful skill with peers.

2. An SLP, midway through his clinical fellowship at a sub-acute rehab facility, evaluates an older gentleman with moderate expressive aphasia and spastic dysarthria. Staff report that he spends days alone without socializing with other residents. The clinical fellow creates three goals for the patient including (1) increased intelligibility when reading sentences, (2) production of adequate vocal quality when sustaining "ah" for 10 seconds, and (3) increased accuracy in picture naming of kitchen and school items.

3. A graduate clinician administers a standardized test to a 4-year-old child. She notes that the child is unable to use negatives appropriately in sentences. She uses the wording of the standardized test item verbatim to formulate the treatment goal.

4. A beginning clinical fellow conducts a bedside swallowing evaluation on an 85-year-old woman in the advanced stages of Alzheimer's dementia. The patient's daughter expresses concerns about her mother's lack of oral intake. After the evaluation, the SLP writes a goal for the patient to demonstrate safe swallowing of restricted consistencies (puree with honey-thick liquids) during three meals per day.

5. A graduate clinician evaluates a 2-year-old dual language learner who is not speaking in either language. Based on the supervisor's advice, the graduate clinician recommends that the parents choose one language for the child to minimize any confusion with language development. The graduate clinician then writes a goal to work on requesting preferred items with gestures and words in only one language.

In the above scenarios, clinicians conducted and analyzed assessments, gathered client-centered information, and identified areas of need. What they failed to do, however, was to synthesize the data to devise functional, impactful goals. As illustrated by these examples, novice clinicians often have difficulty prioritizing skills, generalizing test performance to a larger skillset, choosing goals that are relevant to a specific client's environment and social settings, and factoring the client's diagnosis/prognosis into the plan.

What distinguishes expert clinicians from novices is not necessarily a difference in data collection. Rather, expert clinicians have internalized clinical reasoning processes that allow them to thoughtfully consider and weigh the data in order to formulate functional, meaningful goals.

Sound easy? We fully acknowledge that it is not. This resource guide aims to teach novice speech-language pathologists how to use their knowledge and clinical skills like an expert. Specifically, this guide makes explicit the unseen reasoning and processing that is required to make service delivery personable and functional for all patients. The skill set involved in clinical reasoning enables us to practice at the top of our license.

As you progress through this resource, we encourage you to reflect on:

- where you find yourself getting stuck in the goal-writing process;
- the types and quality of goals you write; and
- ways to improve and strengthen your goal-writing skills to meet your patients' needs.

A Useful Analogy

We all love a good brownie. Pretty much anyone can pick up a box of brownie mix from the grocery store and follow the recipe. It is not necessary to understand the components that are provided in the box. A novice, an individual with little to no experience in baking, will follow the recipe explicitly without deviating from instructions. In fact, failure to do so (e.g., adding less oil or no eggs), could result in an inedible rock.

Over time, a novice baker develops an understanding of the ingredients as separate parts to include knowing what is essential and non-negotiable in the process. This individual also learns which ingredients can be supplemented or improved to take brownies to the next level. Some options include: using part buttermilk and part whole milk, doubling the vanilla, or adding cherries, chocolate chips, or nuts. Experience drives the transition from novice brownie-maker to expert brownie creator.

Let us extend this concept to apply to the skillset of clinical reasoning in speech-language pathology. As speech-language pathologists, treatment goals are our brownies. In the beginning, novice clinicians are given specific "recipes," which they follow without deviation, for both diagnostics and treatment planning. As clinicians' knowledge and experience with patients, settings, and disorder types grow, so does the depth of clinical reasoning skills needed to efficiently create meaningful treatment goals.

One common misconception is that an expert's clinical reasoning skills correlate directly with time or years of experience, but this is not always the case! While it is unnecessary to provide a comprehensive review on this topic, we would like to highlight a few pertinent points that differentiate experts from novices. These points will be useful while reading this text.

- Academic knowledge: Didactic knowledge is a strength for novice clinicians because it is both current and fresh; however, there is less depth to that knowledge. Because of experience, experts are able to efficiently draw from and apply knowledge of relevant content areas when composing treatment goals.

■ Clinical experience: Although it may seem obvious, it is important to acknowledge that novices lack the experience that comes only with patient care. Experts use their wealth of experiences over a career to inform the diagnostic and goal-writing process in their specific work setting.

■ Flexibility: Unlike novices, experts are adept at modifying goals when new information or data are presented. They can efficiently use their academic/continuing education knowledge with clinical experience when incorporating new information so that goals are more functional for the patient.

So how do these differences reveal themselves in expert and novice clinicians with regard to the goal-writing process? To help highlight some pertinent differences, we provide a case study of an adult with a fluency disorder. After the case study, we will operationally define terminology that is key to understanding the clinical reasoning process for expert and novice

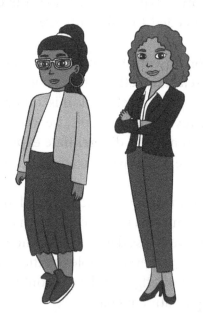

clinicians. While definitions can be dry, they are necessary for understanding the goal-writing process. Do not stop reading at the definitions because, following each definition, we provide differences between the expert and novice clinician from the case study in order to illustrate each concept.

An Introductory Case Study

An 18-year-old college freshman asks to be evaluated and treated at the university speech-language pathology clinic. According to his intake summary, he reports having stuttered his entire life. He has received speech-language pathology services on and off since the age of three. During his school years, he felt comfortable and well supported by teachers, peers, and support staff. He is currently enrolled in a core requirement, a public speaking course, where he is required to give impromptu, timed speeches that will be graded. He wants to achieve an A in the course without accommodation. Evaluation results include:

- a severity equivalent of moderate on the Stuttering Severity Instrument (SSI-4; Riley & Bakker, 2009);
- a mild-moderate impact rating on the Overall Assessment of the Speaker's Experience of Stuttering (OASES; Yaruss & Quesal, 2016); and
- secondary characteristics while speaking including eye blinks and facial grimaces.

A Novice Clinician's Response

"I think this client would benefit from easy onset, relaxation, and breathing exercises. I can see adapting materials from 'turtle talk' to demonstrate slow rate and bumpy versus smooth speech."

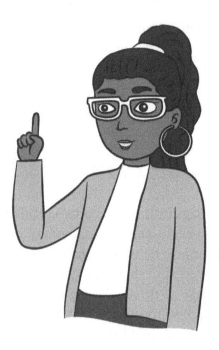

Proposed Goals

1. The client will identify bumpy versus smooth speech in 90% of opportunities.

2. When provided a model, the client will use easy onset at the word-phrase level in 90% of opportunities.

3. When provided a model, the client will use easy onset at the sentence level in 90% of opportunities.

4. During a structured therapy session, the client will imitate common age-appropriate sayings using smooth speech in 8 of 10 trials.

5. The client will self-report 90% accuracy during a home program on diaphragmatic breathing.

6. The client will demonstrate 100% fluent speech during a 10-minute interaction.

An Experienced Clinician's Response

"The important factors to consider include this client's quality of life from the OASES, the required speeches in class, the secondary behaviors he is exhibiting, and the client's personal goals. This client is not new to stuttering; he has a long history of speech therapy so it is safe to assume that he has foundational knowledge of fluency shaping and stuttering modification techniques. We need to have a follow-up conversation about the client's preferences and self-perceived successes. The focus of therapy should be functional application of therapeutic strategies to enhance the client's self-perceived success in a classroom setting."

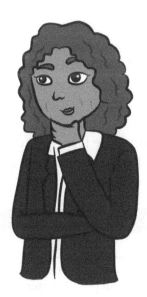

Proposed Goals

1. The client will demonstrate the use of fluency shaping or stuttering modification strategies at least 10 times during a two-minute structured conversation on a topic of the client's choice.

2. Upon viewing a five-minute recording of himself delivering a simulated class speech, the client will identify and discuss with 90% accuracy contexts where his secondary behaviors occur.

3. During a simulated three-minute class presentation to an unfamiliar listener, the client will independently use fluency shaping or stuttering modification strategies at least 15 times.

4. Before speaking activities in a classroom setting, the client will use a self-disclosure statement about stuttering a minimum of two times in three weeks as evidenced by self-report.

Terminology in Clinical Reasoning

Prototypes

In the medical literature, the term 'prototypes' is often referred to as 'illness scripts'. Prototypes are the clinician's background

Table 1–1. Prototype: Case Study Application

Novice	Expert
This clinician is using a prototype of a textbook stuttering case (e.g., a young child who is brought to a private therapy setting by his parents for fluency therapy). She uses her limited fluency prototypes to approach treatment planning for the adult in this case study.	Functionality, client characteristics, and the client's goals inform which prototype is referenced. The expert clinician in this case study is working with the prototype of an adult client living with a fluency disorder who needs functional strategies and goals in his current situation and context (i.e., a university course).

knowledge, domain-specific knowledge, or internal database of characteristics associated with particular diagnoses (Ginsberg et al., 2016; Harjai & Tiwari, 2009, p. 306).

Logic

It is essential to acknowledge logic in the clinical reasoning process. Logic, in simplified terms, is the process by which an individual reaches a conclusion. Researchers who study how clinicians make decisions in healthcare settings have found that experts and novices differ in their use of logic (Shin, 2019). The two types discussed in the literature are inductive and deductive logic.

- Inductive reasoning, or data-driven logic, is a type of logic where the clinician examines all the information that has been gathered and then draws a conclusion based on those facts. The clinician forms a hypothesis only after considering the information as a whole, which includes the patient's history, environment, etc. This approach can be thought of as a "forward" logic process.
- Deductive reasoning, or hypothesis-driven logic, is a type of logic where the clinician first considers established mental models (i.e., prototypes) to solve the problem and then reaches a solution based on the most relevant prototype. This approach can be thought of as a backward logic process.

There is no correct type of logic in patient care. Rather, expert clinicians are able to use both types of logic flexibly and efficiently during the diagnostic and treatment planning

Table 1–2. Logic: Case Study Application	
Novice	*Expert*
The novice clinician is using deductive reasoning. The goals are derived primarily from the patient diagnosis (fluency disorder). The clinician immediately jumps to known interventions such as an introduction to "easy onset," which in this case is inappropriate for a young adult who needs help with skills related to his college course. The client has a prior history of therapy and likely has already been taught "easy onset." As stated previously, the novice clinician has few prototypes to use for making clinical decisions and client-centered goals so her deductive reasoning is largely ineffective.	The expert considers patient-specific and clinical information as a whole—diagnosis, case history, patient's experiences, preferences—prior to drawing conclusions and developing meaningful goals (inductive reasoning). Although she likely has a number of prototypes to choose from, she is not limited by them. Again, expert clinicians are more flexible in their ability to use both types of logic as the situation arises (Shin, 2019). Even when an expert may not have many prototypes for a certain client or patient, the expert is more likely to prioritize patient and setting factors to arrive at clinical decisions that address the individual's needs.

processes. Novice clinicians may limit themselves to one type of logic at a time to the potential detriment of the client.

Clinician Factors

This term includes both contextual factors and cognitive factors (Huhn et al., 2011). Contextual factors are a clinician's stored patient prototypes related to their clinical experience, life circumstances and personal experiences, and social-emotional characteristics. Cognitive factors relate to a clinician's critical thinking abilities (i.e., use of logic) and their judgment. Every clinician will bring the depth and breadth of his/her own knowledge and experience to patient care.

Table 1–3. Clinician Factors: Case Study Application

Novice	*Expert*
The novice clinician demonstrates her lack of experience with this population by jumping directly to treatments that are inappropriate for the client. Her knowledge is evidence-based and current but solely based on didactic experiences (i.e., what she has learned in class). Although she has personal knowledge about the relevant context (a college classroom), she fails to leverage her contextual knowledge to inform this client's plan of care.	The expert clinician demonstrates a broad base of knowledge with which to approach this case. She appreciates both the disorder and the patient's circumstances (college student), and she brings a level of maturity to her thinking observed in her sound logic and recognition of knowledge gaps (e.g., the need for follow-up conversations). The clinician leverages both contextual and cognitive factors in her reasoning.

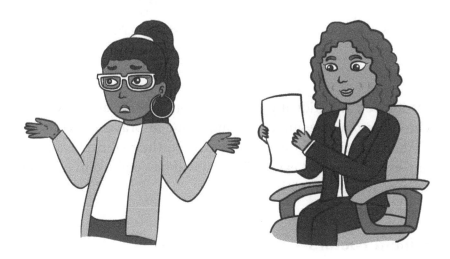

Setting Factors

SLPs work in diverse settings each with unique demands related to environmental characteristics, frequency and duration of service delivery, and demands by third parties (i.e., health

Table 1–4. Setting Factors: Case Study Application	
Novice	*Expert*
Novice clinicians have limited experiences and exposure to the profession as a whole resulting in difficulty accounting for and integrating practice guidelines, environmental characteristics, service delivery constraints, and third-party requirements. In the case study, the novice clinician does not recognize the contribution of setting factors in treatment planning such as characteristics of a college environment or the frequency and duration of therapy within a reasonable timeframe,etc. She may need to acknowledge that her scope of practice for a client with this disorder is not sufficient.	The expert clinician focuses clinical decisions on self-acceptance and self-advocacy, which is essential when treating fluency disorders in patients (ASHA's practice guidelines: "Developing culturally and linguistically relevant intervention plans focused on helping the individual achieve more fluent speech and self-acceptance of dysfluency, providing treatment, documenting progress, and determining appropriate dismissal criteria." [ASHA, n.d.-a]). This clinician proposes goals within a college setting that can be achieved in a realistic timeframe.

insurance). Additionally, setting factors include an individual clinician's practice guidelines and scope of practice according to their training. For example, based on their clinical training and experience, not every clinician will be qualified to provide therapy for vented patients.

Patient Factors

Making appropriate clinical decisions involves taking patient factors into consideration. Patient factors include social-emotional characteristics and, most importantly, the client's personal goals for treatment (Nobriga & St. Clair, 2018). Patient factors also include individual performance during evaluation/assessments, medical and rehabilitation history, abilities

Table 1–5. Patient Factors: Case Study Application

Novice	Expert
In this case study, the novice clinician neglects the client's life experiences/goals (e.g., prior history therapy, performance in class). Even when considering certain client factors (e.g., "age-appropriate sayings"), she does not connect the data, disorder prototype, and the client's life circumstances to write functional goals. The fluency disorder and goal of fluent speech are the primary determinants in treatment planning, and she largely disregards patient factors in her clinical decision.	The expert clinician capitalizes on information provided by the client and assessment results to identify data that are important to clinical goal setting. For this expert clinician, the diagnosis is actually secondary to the patient factors. For example, the clinician is highlighting the client's personal goal of increasing success in the classroom. Specifically, she prioritizes the client's score on the OASES—which provides information on quality of life— over his score on the SSI-4.

and experiences, and developmental and educational skills. Patient factors are one of the three critical components of evidence-based practice (EBP) in which the clinician integrates clinical expertise/expert opinion, external evidence, and the patient/caregiver perspective to provide high quality services for patients and their families (ASHA, n.d.-b). In a person-family centered approach, some of the benefits include improved clinical decision making and person-centered goals which result in better implementation of evidence-based practice in treatment (ASHA, n.d.-c).

Clinical Reasoning

We have now arrived at the meat and potatoes of this resource guide: clinical reasoning. This term is defined differently depending on where you look in the literature. In medicine, for example, clinical reasoning is described in terms of the cognitive skills underlying the differential diagnostic process: recognizing patterns, using intuition, weighing probabilities, utilizing dynamic analysis, comparing and contrasting illness scripts, and being aware of biases and faulty heuristics (Richards et al., 2020; Schuwirth et al., 2020; Thampy et al., 2019). Physicians concentrate on the diagnostic process because it leads directly to a specific medication or surgery to remediate the problem. In the field of speech-language pathology and allied health more broadly, the diagnostic process is only the first step of a longer process. SLPs identify the problem and then devise an individualized plan to address that problem in the larger context of the individual's life. Although clinical reasoning underlies both the diagnostic and goal-planning process, our intent is to focus on the latter.

For the purposes of this text, we have devised our own working definition of clinical reasoning in goal writing that can

Table 1–6. Clinical Reasoning: Case Study Application

Novice	*Expert*
When engaging in clinical reasoning, the novice clinician does not effectively synthesize assessment data or devise viable treatment options based on the evaluation. As stated earlier, she relies on her available prototype to create goals.	The expert efficiently sorts through all the available data, highlights specific information such as the client's self-perceptions, secondary behaviors, and the client's goal of achieving an A grade, and makes treatment decisions based on the age and experience of the client. She considers treatment options for addressing fluency more directly, but ultimately opts for approaches that prioritize the client's situational needs.

be learned and then practiced. Clinical reasoning is the complex cognitive process that uses deductive and inductive reasoning to synthesize relevant clinician, setting, and patient factors through the lens of person- and family-centered care. An essential first step is that the SLP uses assessment data to reach a diagnosis, which then initiates the goal-planning process. There are two processes that occur at this stage. First, the SLP synthesizes clinician, setting, and patient factors. Second, the SLP connects evaluation data with viable treatment options. Ultimately the combination of these processes, along with the use of forward and backward logic, results in meaningful, patient-centered treatment goals. BROWNIES!

Goal Concept

We have created this term to acknowledge the early stage of goal planning. Goal concepts are essentially proto-goals, or the general direction in which to proceed. Through goal concepts, clinicians identify areas on which to focus therapy efforts that will impact the client's life. Over time, goal concepts evolve into long- or short-term goals.

Table 1–7. Goal Concept: Case Study Application

Novice	Expert
The novice clinician seems to miss the client's concerns. Goal concepts are difficult to identify; her objectives inadequately address the client's goal of giving a class presentation and they ignore his psychosocial needs.	The expert's objectives all fall under one goal concept: for the client to successfully deliver a presentation in class.

Table 1–8. Treatment Goals: Case Study Application	
Novice	*Expert*
The novice's goals adhere to the framework she was taught by instructors and/or clinical mentors. She demonstrates a familiarity with the criteria for writing goals but is inflexible in their application. The goals she has written are not relevant to the patient's current needs in this situation and attainability is questionable. For example, some goals work at the level of isolation (i.e., word and sentence level), whereas the last goal targets fluency in spontaneous speech during a 10-minute conversation.	Goals are written by integrating the setting and patient factors to address present and future needs. Goals are not formulaic in nature, but rather are written to promote optimal functionality in a realistic manner. For example, each goal is measured in accordance with the skill being demonstrated and/ or utilized rather than by correct or incorrect trials.

Treatment Goals

As you have undoubtedly learned, treatment goals are statements written for or in collaboration with the client as a blueprint for measuring habilitative or rehabilitative progress. Well-written treatment goals include the following criteria: they are measurable, achievable/attainable, specific, relevant, and time-bound.

Conclusion

We have finished defining the individual components involved in clinical reasoning that are required to write meaningful goals (e.g., logic, prototypes, patient factors, etc.). By providing contrasting examples of how novices and experts approach goal writing, we have attempted to illustrate how each component contributes to the process (and how goals can be ineffective if they are not taken into account). When a novice starts her journey as an SLP, she typically brings an incomplete understanding of each component, which in turn impacts clinical reasoning for both diagnostic and treatment processes. Experts not only understand the required components, but they efficiently and flexibly apply them with the individual patient as the priority. We fully acknowledge that moving from novice to expert in goal writing takes time and practice.

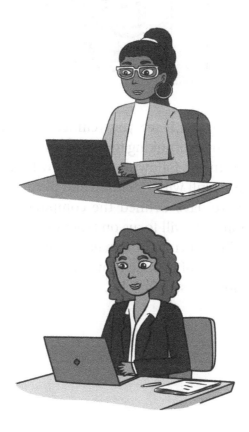

Be patient with this journey. Establishing new or correcting old reasoning skills will take time and intentionality; however,

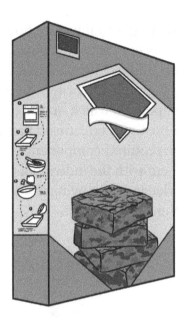

with practice you WILL see your clinical reasoning abilities transition from novice thinking to expert reasoning. The framework presented in the following chapters will help you tackle and focus on this skill with intention and purpose.

Now that we have defined the components involved in clinical reasoning, we will focus on types of data that influence goal selection. To return to our analogy, we have defined what goes into the process of making brownies. We next consider key ingredients before we start baking.

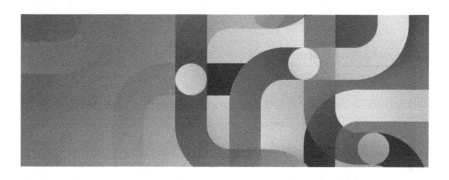

2 Goal Framework

Key Questions

Picture this—it is a cold, rainy day. Your favorite music is playing in the background and the lighting is perfect. You are in the mood to bake, and brownies are on the menu. You open the pantry to pull out the ingredients and see all the options and possibilities for your brownies. To begin preparations for baking, you pull out all possible ingredients without a specific recipe in mind. In our analogy, the ingredients you will be using are the data you will be collecting and working with to create patient-centered goals.

In this section, we will briefly describe the types of data typically gathered by category, which may or may not be used in goal writing (e.g., depending on setting or patient population). For the purposes of this resource, we describe common types of data, indicate where these data are commonly found, and highlight differences across medical and educational settings. The data types are categorized by three questions: Who is the patient? What is the patient's current communication/swallowing status? and, What is important to the patient and his/her family? These questions align directly with the International Classification of Functioning, Disability and Health (ICF), the framework used by the World Health Organization for measuring and classifying health and disability in individuals (WHO, n.d.).

As you review this chapter, flexibility and perspective are important. We present examples of the types of data collected under each question and encourage you to adapt the information to your specific setting and patient population.

Who Are They?

Medical Information

Description

An essential ingredient in the goal-writing process includes collecting medical diagnoses, comorbidities, medications, allergies, hearing and vision status, maternal health and birth history, feeding/swallowing history, diet restrictions, mobility limitations, significant medical events such as illnesses, injuries and surgeries, and previous history of therapies.

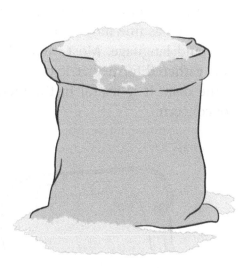

Where It Is Found

This information is typically found in patients' medical records, case history forms, and referral documentation. It may be obtained through records available onsite, patient disclosure, or clinician-initiated records requests.

Differences Across Settings

Access to medical history may be more limited in educational settings as compared to medical settings.

Developmental Information

Description

This ingredient is essential in some settings and optional in others. It describes the patient's achievement of developmental milestones in areas such as fine motor, gross motor, cognitive skills, and speech and language. Most often, developmental appropriateness is gathered for pediatric clients to be used as functional baseline data. It is useful in the identification of potential areas of concern.

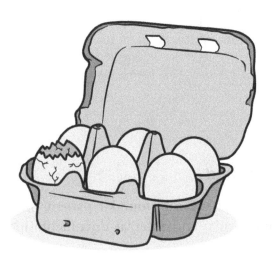

Where It Is Found

This is most often collected from caregivers or parents via an in-person or virtual interaction and/or a client case history form.

Differences Across Settings

Developmental data are often collected in both medical and educational settings; however, the interpretation of these data may differ. In the educational setting, the interpretation aids in decision-making, whereas in medical settings developmental data inform functional status for treatment and justification of services. Developmental data are typically not relevant for patients past adolescence.

Educational Information

Description

Similar to developmental information, this ingredient varies in its importance in the recipe relative to the age of the patient. For pediatric patients, this type of data provides the potential functional impact of communication deficits on the ability to function and thrive within a learning environment. For adult patients, it provides insight into an individual's level of education to inform literacy and language use, and vocational or occupational training.

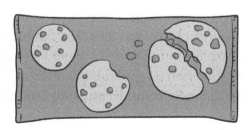

Where It Is Found

These data are obtained as part of a client's case history form. Information can be retrieved from the referral source (parent and/or teacher), but also through in-person interactions with patients and caregivers.

Differences Across Settings

Educational information is gathered in both medical and educational settings; however, the roles these data play vary within each setting. Academic need within educational settings is the purpose for the referral and is also necessary for the qualification of services in most educational settings. Educational information serves as the point of reference and framework for establishing treatment plans should a client show educational impact relative to his/her speech and language deficits. Within medical settings, this information can assist with diagnostic and treatment-based decisions.

Language Experience

Description

Language experience refers to someone's exposure and use of language(s) and dialects. This will be especially important if a person is exposed to and speaks more than one language. When considering a child, language exposure includes data such as age of acquisition of each language and input and output observed in each language from birth. For an adult, language experience information may refer to the percentage of input and output of each language spoken on a regular basis. Having this information will inform diagnostic and treatment planning in terms of which language to conduct initial assessments, treatment, and home programming.

Where It Is Found

Information related to language experience for children or adults can be gathered through informative structured question- naires. Some examples for children include the Bilingual Input Output Survey (BIOS) which is part of the Bilingual English Spanish Assessment (BESA, Pena et al., 2018) or the Alberta Language and Development Questionnaire (ALDeQ; Paradis et al., 2010). For adults, this information can be gathered by asking during the patient interview which languages are spoken to the patient and in which languages the patient responds. Patient self-report for language dominance and the amount of each language used throughout the day has been found to be a reliable measure related to language abilities in each language. In addition, standardized tools such as the Language Proficiency Questionnaire (LEAP-Q; Marian et al., 2009) may be used with adult populations.

Differences Across Settings

It is important in any setting to take into consideration the lan- guage experience of the patient (pediatric or adult). These data can have a significant impact on services provided in the educa- tional and medical settings. With half of the world's population speaking more than one language, these data are pertinent to diagnostic and treatment planning.

- Educational Setting: Information related to language experience may have an impact on educational place- ment recommendations (e.g., dual language versus monolingual classroom). Further, the Multi-Tiered System of Support (MTSS) would also be impacted by the child's language experience; the SLP would need to know which language(s) the child would benefit from when targeting areas of concern.

▪ Medical Setting: Information related to language experience would be beneficial to help treatment planning, and to educate other professionals about the patient's preferred language for health care contexts. For example, some patients may benefit from communication boards in another language while others may have a preference for which language is used in specific settings.

What Is Their Current Communication and Swallowing Status?

Diagnostic Assessments

Description

Performance measures are a critical part of the data clinicians use for diagnostic decisions that in turn inform goal concepts. Common performance measures are standardized or criterion-referenced instruments that assess an area of concern for the patient (e.g., communication, cognition). Performance measures may also be naturalistic or qualitative such as a language or reading sample from the patient, which can be compared to a normative sample or used to measure progress over time. In addition, qualitative measures can include dynamic assessment and observation assessment that provide information regarding the client's learning potential and current level of functioning. Performance on dynamic assessment measures may also inform the use of evidence-based intervention methods during treatment, which should be considered when creating patient goals. For example, if a patient with dysarthria responds well to overexaggerating his articulation during dynamic assessment, this will inform treatment planning and goal writing.

Where It Is Found

A clinician will find this information in the patient's assessment records, specifically test protocols or forms. Interpretation of performance measures and recommendations are also commonly provided as part of the diagnostic report.

Differences Across Settings

- Educational Settings: In an educational setting, a student's score on a performance measure must show an educational need in order to receive speech and language services. Performance measures relative to a student's language skills inform education specific goals.
- Medical Settings: In health care settings, scores on performance measures must show medical necessity and functional need during activities of daily living for speech-language services. These areas must be reflected in the patient's treatment plan and can be influenced by third-party payers.

Diagnostic Decisions

Description

After the assessments have been administered and analyzed, the clinician then engages in the differential diagnostic process and forms clinical impressions. This process is comprehensive and multi-faceted and will likely include medical, developmental, educational, language experience, and performance measures. For the scope of this resource, we will not provide additional details on this process, but the importance and value of diagnostic decisions are paramount to treatment planning and goal writing.

Where It Is Found

These data are the result of the diagnostic process and are found in the clinician's interpretation of assessments.

Differences Across Settings

Although the purpose, outcomes, and plan of care that result from these decisions will vary (i.e., educational need versus functional impact on daily living), this information is foundational regardless of setting.

What Is Important to Them?

Environment

Description

Patient data are essential ingredients in goal writing that refer to the various communicative settings in which a client lives and participates. Environments can include schools, homes, social settings, workplaces, community locations, and all of the people in those settings. It may also be necessary to consider current environments as well as ones in the future, such as for a patient that will soon be discharged home from a rehabilitation facility.

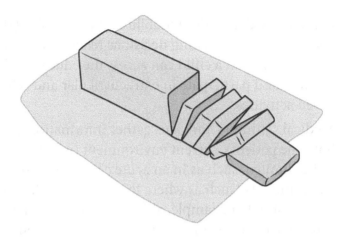

Where It Is Found

Data about the client's environment are typically gathered during interviews with family members, caregivers, and the clients themselves, and can also be found in case history forms or standardized tools. For example, the Assessment for Living With Aphasia, Second Edition (Kagan et al., 2013) includes questions about the individual's social networks and participation in personally-relevant environments.

Differences Across Settings

Although information about a client's environments must be incorporated in any clinical setting when devising goals, there are also key differences between educational and medical settings.

- Educational settings: When considering educational environments, particularly those in a traditional school setting, the client's educational needs in relation to the child's ability to learn and participate in the least restrictive environment determine qualification for services and where and when services are provided. The principles of the Individuals with Disability Education Act (IDEA, 2004) direct goal-writing decisions related to service provision so that a child can access the educational curriculum and participate in extracurricular and school-based activities.

- Medical settings: Clinicians gather information about both the patient's current environment (which may be rather limited, such as in an acute care unit) and future environments (such as where the patient would like to participate). For example, although home with family is the current environment for meals, a future environment might include the patient's favorite restaurant prior to his motor vehicle accident. Careful consideration of environments in goal writing is directly related to an individual's quality of life in accordance with the ICF model. In the medical setting, goals should be written to help the patient participate in chosen activities across different environments, which will impact their long-term health and well-being.

Interests/Life Events

Description

Although communicative environments are difficult to separate from this category, interests and life events will include specific activities or tasks (e.g., a role in a school play, a book club discussion), psychological well-being (e.g., feeling confident when interacting with peers, being unafraid when swallowing thin liquids), and academic or social achievements (e.g., a passing grade on an English assignment, participating in a group game on the playground). This category includes past, present, and future interests and/or life events.

Where It Is Found

Similar to environments, a list of the client's interests are generally gathered from written or oral case histories.

Differences Across Settings

This information is typically collected in both medical and educational settings.

Patient and Family Priorities

Description

This ingredient is non-negotiable because there is a correlation between the perceived value of therapy services and participation in the therapeutic process (i.e., buy-in). The best-written plan of care will not be relevant or even impactful if the individual's and family members' preferences are not taken into account. These preferences may include but are not limited to religious, cultural, and social domains.

It is important to recognize that expressed priorities may not always address what is necessary to accomplish in therapy; however, they should always be incorporated in some way. For example, a 13-year-old student would likely not prioritize the use of age-appropriate syntax to support his academic performance but would prioritize being able to converse with friends at lunch. In another example, a spouse might express a desire that her husband with expressive aphasia speak like he used to; this priority could be shaped into devising and reciting a four-minute speech at his daughter's wedding. A final example: a grandmother's priority for her 8-year-old grandson may be to recite a prayer in front of a group during a religious service. Just as the child's siblings have done in the past, he might choose to practice a short prayer during a small group activity or family meal.

Where It Is Found

Initially, this information is included in case history forms. This initial impression can then be expanded upon during semi-structured interviews. SLPs may choose to provide options for clients or ask guided questions rather than open-ended questions (e.g., "Is it important for you to be heard in public-speaking events without feeling vocal strain" versus "What is your goal in voice therapy?"). These responses can progress to more specific patient priorities as rapport is established between the patient and clinician.

Differences Across Settings

Although patient/family member priorities may be incorporated in different ways, there are no important distinctions between educational and medical settings.

Conclusion

Now that we have identified and organized our ingredients, it is time to bake. Fudgy brownies, brownies with nuts, cake brownies, or blonde brownies—what to choose when they all sound delicious? It is time to commit to a brownie recipe (chocolate fudge brownies, of course). With a recipe in mind, you eliminate unnecessary ingredients and then add the key ingredients for the batter to the mixing bowl. Once all ingredients are in the bowl, it is time to start the mixing process.

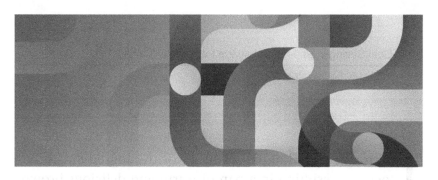

3 Goal Framework Guide

Drumroll Please

The magic of baking is when all of the ingredients come together resulting in a pan of warm and delicious brownies. Once the ingredients are measured according to the recipe, they are added together in the mixing bowl. The act of stirring combines the ingredients into a cohesive batter, which is then baked into the final product.

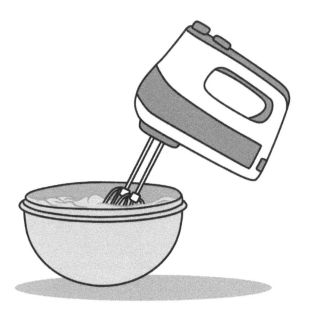

As clinicians, we follow a similar procedure when proceeding from diagnostic information to formulating treatment goals and plans. The exact process and specific ingredients vary according to each individual patient. Patient and environmental information used in the clinical reasoning process may be ordered or prioritized differently to create relevant, meaningful goals for a specific individual. For beginning clinicians, effort and attention to each step is necessary to learn the processing framework. With practice and repetition, the recipe/cognitive process is memorized, and the recipe is relied on less and less. On the other hand, we think it is important to acknowledge that no matter a clinician's career stage, the goal-writing process is intentional and challenging.

Now to introduce a basic framework for crafting meaningful, patient-centered goals. Figure 3–1 illustrates the phases of

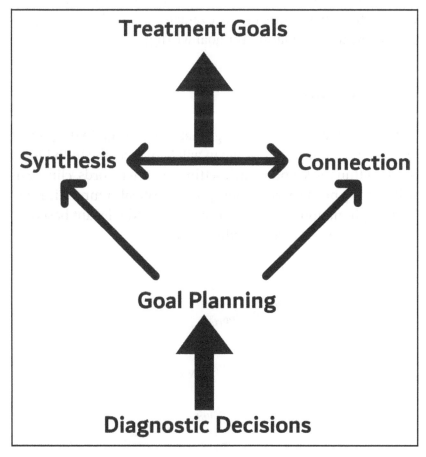

Figure 3–1. Clinical reasoning.

goal-writing. We wish to emphasize the fluidity of this process; once the diagnostic decision has been made, other phases do not necessarily occur chronologically.

Goal-Writing Framework

Diagnostic Decision

A diagnostic decision is determined based on assessments and other data gathered during the evaluation. The diagnostic process forms the foundation for goal writing.

Goal Planning

This phase starts by considering what is important to the patient and family, and how the clinician will help meet the individual's needs within the scope of each setting. In other words, clinicians will identify primary goal concepts (e.g., social communication, healthy phonation) which are functional and relevant based on the setting (medical versus educational).

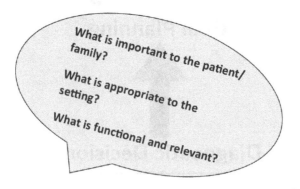

Synthesis

In this phase, the clinician uses inductive reasoning to disregard data that are irrelevant, highlight data that are meaningful, and then combine the essential data in support of the goal concept. At the end of this phase, the clinician has better conceptualized the goal, but it is still incomplete in form.

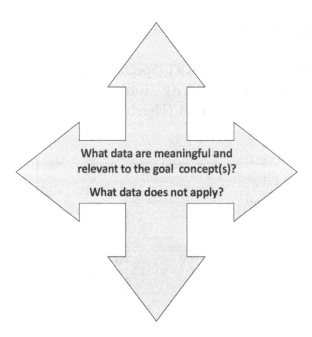

What data are meaningful and relevant to the goal concept(s)?

What data does not apply?

Connection

In this phase, the clinician uses deductive reasoning to consider treatment options (e.g., evidence-based treatments, indirect approaches) for targeting each identified goal concept. The approach that is selected is used to construct a purposeful, measurable goal.

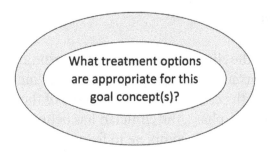

Treatment Goals

Well-written goals are SMART (Specific, Measurable, Accessible, Realistic, and Time-bound; e.g., Torres, 2013), but more importantly, they are SMARTER (Hersh et al., 2012; Figure 3–2).

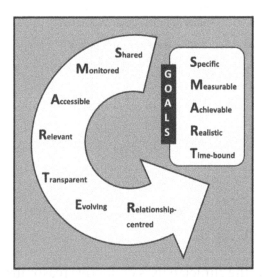

Figure 3–2. SMARTER goals. *Source*: Hersh, D., Worrall, L., Howe, T., Sherratt, S., and Davidson, B. (2012). *SMARTER* goal setting in aphasia rehabilitation. *Aphasiology*, *26*(2), 220–233. https://doi.org/10.1080/02687 038.2011.640392 © Taylor & Francis. Reproduced with permission of the Licensor through PLSclear.

SMART describes the nature of goals, whereas SMARTER emphasizes the context (i.e., the patient's life) in which goals are written. The SMARTER framework encourages clinicians to work collaboratively with patients and family members to create not only measurable but meaningful goals for the individual.

- Shared: collaborative input from personally-relevant stakeholders
- Monitored: measurable and reviewed with the client over the course of therapy
- Accessible: understandable to the client to promote participation
- Relevant: functional for the individual's life circumstances
- Transparent: logical and includes sub-goals needed to achieve the primary goal
- Evolving: modifiable and flexible to accommodate the client's changing needs
- Relationship-centered: designed to enhance personal connections with others

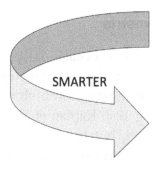

Next, we will illustrate each stage of the goal writing process in two case examples—one medical, one educational—as executed by an expert clinician. Note that the diagnostic decision, which serves as the foundation of the framework, is provided in the case description. In addition to talking through the process, we will highlight some common pitfalls seen in novice clinicians in each phase.

Case Example 1: Theo

Who Are They?

Medical Information

Theo is a 58-year-old, English-speaking male with a primary diagnosis of early-onset dementia of the Alzheimer variant. His neurologist notes that symptoms are consistent with early to mid stage of disease progression.

What Is Their Current Communication and Swallowing Status?

Diagnostic Assessments

Although he complains of occasional problems with word-retrieval, this is not observed in spontaneous speech during the evaluation. Assessment results show high naming scores (57/60 on the Boston Naming Test; Kaplan et al., 2001). His language skills are strong overall, but he exhibits moderate to severe deficits in executive functioning (moderate to severe range on the Cognitive-Linguistic Quick Test, CLQT; Helm-Estabrooks,

2001). In particular, tasks that involve organization, planning, and higher-level executive functioning are challenging.

Diagnostic Decisions

According to assessment results, Theo presents with mild-moderate cognitive-communication deficits due to dementia. Based on the nature of the disease, the clinician recognizes that Theo's underlying impairments will continue to impact his daily interactions, social engagement, and participation in activities of daily living.

What Is Important to Them?

Interests /Life Events

His previous occupation was electrical engineering. Due to his diagnosis, he is unable to work, although he reports a desire to return to his job. He exhibits difficulty reading long texts and can no longer drive. He has a supportive wife and 16-year-old daughter. His social life and environments have shrunk and consist primarily of immediate family and home.

Environment

Theo is aware that his daughter prefers to talk to her mother rather than to him and this hurts his feelings. He states that he has no purpose other than to sit at home, watch TV, and occasionally walk the dog. His spouse reports that he cannot be relied upon to feed the pets or take his medications. Social events are challenging because he is unable to keep up with fast-paced conversations, particularly in noisy environments, and he is unable to maintain the topic of conversation. His wife expresses embarrassment about his long, meandering conversations with others, but Theo is largely unaware that his social interaction skills are not well received. In general, Theo is unable to recognize his deficits or their impact on his loved ones.

Patient and Family Priorities

The family is requesting help in navigating Theo's communication challenges and establishing ways for them to continue being socially active.

Goal Planning

Goal Concept One

Maintaining the ability to socialize with family and close friends is a priority for the couple. Improving social interaction is identified as an important goal concept so that Theo can preserve important relationships in his life.

Goal Concept Two

Since Theo is no longer able to work, he is struggling to fill his time with purposeful activities that he can manage independently. This goal concept involves modifying the environment so that Theo can be successful in chosen activities of daily living, which could also include new activities.

Common Novice Pitfalls

1. A novice clinician might wish to support Theo's desire to return to work by creating a goal concept about improving work-related skills. Because of Theo's degenerative disease,

this direction would be both frustrating and futile. He has already ceased working, so the focus should be on improving Theo's current environment.

2. A novice clinician may choose to focus on more foundational conversation skills such as turn-taking rather than on Theo's specific challenge—maintaining the topic of conversation—which is negatively affecting his social interactions.

3. A novice clinician may be tempted to target safety skills such as answering basic demographic questions (e.g., name, address, primary care provider) without taking into consideration that his current social circle consists mostly of his immediate family. The focus should be on improving communication with loved ones such as with his daughter.

Synthesis

Goal Concept One: Social Interaction

The clinician utilizes data relevant to social interaction skills, specifically, the ability to maintain the topic of conversation. Language skills are a strength and do not need to be targeted for this goal. Executive functions such as organization, short-term memory, and planning underlie the ability to direct and maintain the topic of conversation so these skills are prioritized. The clinician highlights data regarding Theo's social network and important communication partners such as his wife and daughter.

Goal Concept Two: Environmental Modifications for Activities of Daily Living

For this goal, the clinician again prioritizes the impaired executive functions and lack of self-awareness that are impacting

Theo's independence in chosen daily activities. For example, his memory deficits explain why he fails to regularly feed the family's pets. His language skills are largely irrelevant for this goal concept, but the clinician does consider Theo's reading abilities in order to design appropriate environmental modifications. For this goal concept, the clinician reviews Theo's interests to devise ideas for new, meaningful activities.

Common Novice Pitfalls

1. A novice clinician may prioritize Theo's complaint about occasional word-finding problems. These difficulties are infrequent, and do not affect social interaction as much as his impaired topic maintenance abilities.

2. A novice clinician might overemphasize activities that Theo is already doing such as watching TV and walking the dog. Since Theo is already doing these activities independently, the clinician should focus efforts on expanding environmental supports that increase participation in other purposeful activities.

3. A novice clinician might overprioritize Theo's performance on the CLQT and decide to target tasks in which he did poorly. Focusing on improving short-story recall or mazes will not address Theo's and his family's primary concerns.

Connection

Goal Concept One: Social Interaction

The clinician has recently begun working with this population and is not knowledgeable on current practices for targeting topic maintenance. A quick review of the literature indicates (1) executive functions are typically not directly targeted in the context of neurodegenerative disease, and (2) both visual and auditory external cues have been found to be effective in supporting topic maintenance in patients with early to mid-stage dementia.

Goal Concept Two: Environmental Modifications for Activities of Daily Living

The clinician considers principles of neurorehabilitation with Theo. Specifically, she wants to use the principle of specificity, training in the context of specific, personally relevant activities, to ensure that therapy can generalize to the home environment. She also draws from literature on psychosocial factors that predict positive outcomes in individuals with neurogenic communication disorders. Applied to Theo, therapy efforts that add structure to his environment will help foster Theo's independence and empowerment.

Common Novice Pitfalls

1. A novice clinician might not consider the literature. Instead, she might rely only on personal experiences or knowledge of a related population (e.g., patients with aphasia).

2. A novice clinician might ask co-workers what they have tried in the past, which is not a sufficient substitute for external evidence. However, co-workers' and personal experiences do complement and provide functionality to evidence found in the literature.

3. A novice clinician might choose a strategy that works for her personally such as use of mnemonic devices. Again, anecdotal evidence should not replace scientific evidence as we know from evidence-based practice.

Treatment Goals

The clinician feels that the two goal concepts can be collapsed into one overarching long-term goal: The patient will increase use of compensatory strategies to improve social engagement and participation in chosen activities.

In adherence with the SMARTER framework, the clinician creates two objectives and then asks Theo and his wife for their input.

Short-Term Goal 1: Social Interaction

During a 2-minute conversation, the patient will successfully return to the topic of conversation in five of six trials using external cues from his spouse or the clinician.

Short-Term Goal 2: Environmental Modifications for Activities of Daily Living

The patient and his spouse will devise and adopt three external memory and executive function aids to support activities of daily living per patient or family report.

Common Novice Pitfalls

1. A novice clinician often limits her thinking to the client achieving 80% accuracy (or 8 of 10). In many cases, there are significantly more creative, functional, and meaningful ways to measure an objective (Moore, 2018).
2. A novice clinician may not think to share objectives with her clients. We know that involving clients in their own plan of care is highly motivating and facilitates buy-in to the therapeutic process (Abendroth & Whited, 2021).

Clinical Reasoning Goal Writing Template

Theo

What is important to the patient/family?

What is appropriate to the setting?

What is functional and relevant?

Goal Planning:

Suggestions:
- Maintain relationships with family and close friends by improving social interaction skills
- Modify the environment to support chosen activities of daily living

Synthesis:

Suggestions:
- Relevant:
  - Topic maintenance skills
  - Executive functions / self-awareness that underlie topic maintenance
  - Theo's social network
  - Reading abilities
  - Theo's life interests
- Irrelevant:
  - Language skills (e.g., grammar)
  - Occasional word finding problems
  - Current activities that Theo can already do independently
  - Task performance on the CLQT

What data are meaningful and relevant to the goal concept(s)?

What data does not apply?

What treatment options are appropriate for this goal concept(s)?

Connection:

Suggestions:
- Use of visual and auditory external cues to support topic maintenance
- Employing the principle of specificity to train personally-relevant activities
- Adding structure to the environment to foster Theo's independence

STOP & CONSIDER

What are potential novice pitfalls?

Suggestions:
- Targeting language skills such as occasional word finding problems or performance on specific word finding tasks (CLQT)
- Focusing on activities that Theo can already do independently versus exploring new, meaningful activities
- Prioritizing return to work over improving Theo's current environment
- Focusing on foundational conversational skills such as turn taking versus topic-maintenance
- Prioritizing answering basic demographic questions versus improving meaningful communication
- Relying on anecdotal evidence
- Limiting goal writing to 80% accuracy or other less meaningful standards of measure
- Not sharing objectives with Theo

Goals:

Suggestions:
1. During a 2-minute conversation, the patient will successfully return to the topic of conversation in 5 of 6 trials using external cues from his spouse or the clinician.
2. The patient and his spouse will devise and adopt 3 external memory and executive function aids to support activities of daily living per patient or family report.

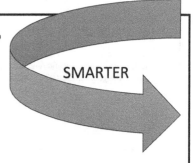

SMARTER

3. As discussed earlier, novice clinicians might write goals that focus on less meaningful, impactful skills. The cause of this common pitfall could be any earlier stage in the goal-writing process: derailed goal concepts, synthesis, or connection.

Case Example 2: Jayden

Who Are They?

Developmental Information

Jayden is a 7-year-old child who is an only child and lives with his mother and father. He was diagnosed with autism at the age of 5 years old. He started using words at 2 years old and uses short sentences to communicate with his parents and caregivers. He reportedly loves Legos and will spend hours in his room constructing intricate buildings. Jayden does not have much social interaction with other children outside of school as he is an only child.

Educational Information and Language Experience

Jayden has been receiving speech and language services in the schools since kindergarten. He is a monolingual English speaker in the second grade. Jayden struggles socially at school due to feeling anxious about how others perceive him, specifically when he feels that someone is upset with him (this information was shared by the school psychologist who is an indirect provider on his IEP). Some examples of events that induce anxiety include when a teacher redirects him or when a friend chooses to do another activity instead of the one that Jayden is doing. In these instances, Jayden does not ask if the person is angry or upset with him; instead he breaks down crying while repeating the phrase "I'm sorry, I'm sorry, I'm sorry." While he can have simple conversations with adults and peers, he exhibits significant difficulty expressing his feelings and he struggles with recognizing and repairing communication breakdowns. His teacher reports that Jayden's academics are significantly impacted by his breakdowns. She states that his frequent breakdowns in the classroom impede his ability to participate with other peers during core learning activities and he has developed few friendships.

What Is Their Current Communication and Swallowing Status?

Diagnostic Assessments

On his most recent reevaluation, he scored within the average to low average range on the PLS-5 (Zimmerman et al., 2011) for both expressive and receptive language. Testing revealed that he has difficulty understanding more abstract language as well as categorizing items, using possessive pronouns, and formulating questions. During a classroom observation Jayden had a breakdown when a friend decided to play on his tablet instead of a board game with Jayden during indoor recess time. Jayden started to cry and repeated "I'm sorry, I'm sorry." This incident lasted 15 minutes and required the teacher and a classroom assistant to help redirect Jayden from his upset state. Ultimately, despite the teacher and the teacher assistant's efforts, Jayden only stopped crying when the bell rang indicating it was time for his class to transition to recess.

Diagnostic Decisions

Jayden presents with a moderate pragmatic language disorder. He scored within the low average range on the Preschool Language Scales, 5th Edition (PLS-5). His academic performance is negatively impacted by his pragmatic and communication challenges as demonstrated by his frequent inability to participate in classroom tasks due to emotional breakdowns. The disruption to his academic participation is the primary justification for his need for intervention.

What Is Important to Them?

Environment

In the home setting, Jayden has fewer anxiety-induced breakdowns than at school. When he has a breakdown at home, his parents have tried putting Jayden in "time away" to calm him down or ignoring this behavior but this often results in an escalation of crying and apologizing similar to at school.

Patient and Family Priorities

Jayden's parents report being concerned about similar anxiety-induced behaviors at home, although breakdowns seem to be far less frequent than at school. They are worried about Jayden's overall social skills. During a recent phone call, his parents disclosed that despite having invited eight children from class, only two came to his birthday party. Jayden cried during and after the party, but was not able to express why he was crying. His parents are seeking additional help from the speech pathologist to see if there are functional goals that can be implemented in his IEP to help with his breakdowns.

Goal Planning

Goal Concept 1

During emotional breakdowns, Jayden is unable to communicate what he is feeling and has difficulty gaining composure to rejoin class activities. An important goal concept for Jayden is to be able to describe his feelings using specific vocabulary during breakdowns so that his communication partner is better able to provide support in the moment.

Goal Concept 2

Jayden's parents and teacher expressed that he does not seek information when he is confused about someone's reactions toward him, which quickly results in breakdowns. This goal concept would help him seek information from a communication partner.

Novice Pitfalls

1. A novice clinician might prioritize areas on the PLS-5 where Jayden performed below average (e.g., figurative language). Goal concepts around understanding metaphors and similes would not be as functional for Jayden as addressing breakdowns that affect his learning time and lead to significant educational impact.

2. A novice clinician might also prioritize increasing socialization and the use of different kinds of social scripts with peers (for example, introducing himself, asking to participate in a game with a peer, etc.). While Jayden may exhibit challenges with social interactions, his difficulties are rooted in his anxiety and misperceptions of how others

respond to and think about him. A more immediate and functional need is Jayden's inability to express how he feels using appropriate vocabulary.

3. A novice clinician may focus on creating symbol systems or social scripts for transitions/breaks, rather than identifying and addressing the communication breakdown.

Synthesis

Goal Concept 1: Using Feelings Vocabulary During Breakdowns

Considering all of the information about Jayden, the clinician prioritizes using feelings and specific vocabulary during breakdowns as this is a critical area that is impacting his ability to participate in the classroom therefore impacting his learning. While he exhibits weaknesses in other areas such as categorizing items and using possessive pronouns, these are not impacting his functional and academic performance. In addition, his diagnosis is a pragmatic versus expressive language disorder.

Goal Concept 2: Seeking Information From a Communication Partner

Seeking information from a communication partner is an important conversational skill and helps to increase pragmatic understanding of a situation. Based on evaluation results, Jayden exhibits difficulties forming questions, which should be targeted functionally. Specifically, his teacher reported that he does not ask questions about others' adverse reactions to him during emotional breakdowns.

Novice Pitfalls

1. A novice clinician might focus on broadly targeting question formulation such as "wh" questions of a picture scene.

2. A novice clinician may prioritize establishing friendships with peers, whereas the academic impact in the classroom with both peers and adults is necessary to address.

3. A novice clinician may focus only on Jayden's identification of emotions in pictures of others. A more appropriate focus is on self-identification in relevant social contexts.

Connection

Goal Concept 1: Using Feeling Vocabulary During Breakdowns

The clinician seeks additional information from the parent and teacher about Jayden's comprehension of feeling vocabulary. The clinician utilizes data obtained from classroom observations to learn more about the environment and context of breakdowns in the classroom. In a search of the literature, the clinician finds the Social-Emotional Learning Intervention (SELF, Poventud et al., 2015) and decides to use portions of the intervention to teach relevant vocabulary.

Goal Concept 2: Seeking Information From a Communication Partner

The clinician references a recent continuing education course in social communication disorders. A review of these references indicates that use of social scripts is an evidence-based method to help children with pragmatic challenges such as Jayden's. The clinician decides that Jayden would benefit from a set of scripted questions that seek information from his communication partners to help with engagement and recall of emotions during breakdowns.

Novice Pitfalls

1. A novice clinician may pull out a workbook that addresses social-emotional communication and may not consider how to individualize the approach for Jayden.

2. A novice clinician may simply pick the most common feeling words (e.g. mad, happy, sad) without taking into consideration parent and teacher input and direct classroom observations. This information would guide the clinician to target applicable feeling vocabulary.

3. A novice clinician likely knows from coursework that the use of scripts is an evidence-based intervention to treat pragmatic challenges. However, a novice may not focus this intervention on Jayden's specific needs (for example, "Why did you _____" or "Are you angry with me?" when he feels anxious or when he is unsure about how people react to him). Instead a novice clinician might use a scripted conversation of a theoretical situation by using pictures available from the internet and formulating more general questions.

Treatment Goals

Jayden's goal areas can be combined into one long-term goal: Jayden will reduce breakdowns in the classroom by increasing his ability to express his feelings and seek information from a communication partner.

In adherence with the SMARTER framework, the clinician creates two objectives and then asks the teacher and parent for their input.

Short-Term Goal 1: Using Feeling Vocabulary During Breakdowns

With the use of a visual aid, Jayden will verbalize a targeted feeling word with a teacher or peer in the classroom in two out of four opportunities in order to decrease frequency of breakdowns.

Short-Term Goal 2: Seeking Information From a Communication Partner

During a structured interaction, Jayden will use a scripted question to seek information from a peer in the classroom (e.g., "Why did you _____?", "Are you ___ with me?") in two out of four opportunities to help reduce anxiety by improving communication.

Novice Pitfalls

1. A novice clinician might write a goal that does not consider the amount of support (i.e., cueing, scaffolding) needed within the classroom environment.

2. A novice clinician may write a goal targeting tangible language skills (i.e., identification of feeling words) instead of considering Jayden's ability to access the academic curriculum and participate in age-appropriate socialization.

3. A novice clinician may write a goal using standard measurements (i.e., 8 out of 10 accuracy) rather than measuring functional application of the skill.

Clinical Reasoning Goal Writing Template

Jayden

Goal Planning:

> Suggestions:
> - Describe feelings using specific vocabulary
> - Seek information from a communication partner

What is important to the patient/family?

What is appropriate to the setting?

What is functional and relevant?

Synthesis:

Suggestions:
- Relevant:
  - ○ Specific vocabulary about feelings during breakdowns
  - ○ Functional question formulation
- Irrelevant:
  - ○ Possessive pronouns, categorizing items, and other language areas
  - ○ Broadly using "wh" questions not related to functional situations

What data are meaningful and relevant to the goal concept(s)?

What data does not apply?

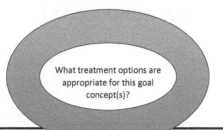

What treatment options are appropriate for this goal concept(s)?

Connection:

Suggestions:
- Adapting a social-emotional learning intervention to teach relevant vocabulary
- Employing use of social scripts to script functional questions for pragmatic purposes

STOP & CONSIDER

What are potential novice pitfalls?

Suggestions:
- Prioritizing standardized assessment tasks over functionality
- Prioritizing social interactions and friendships more generally versus what is academically relevant
- Employing external aids such as picture prompts instead of focusing on social communication
- Considering "wh" questions that are not based on functional context
- Identifying emotions in pictures of others instead of self-identification
- Using workbooks versus individualized treatment methods
- Choosing only common emotion words
- Letting materials guide intervention instead of functional situations
- Writing a goal that doesn't provide sufficient support

Goals:

Suggestions:
1. With the use of a visual aid, Jayden will verbalize a targeted feeling word with a teacher or peer in the classroom in two out of four opportunities in order to decrease frequency of breakdowns.
2. During a structured interaction, Jayden will use a scripted question to seek information from a peer in the classroom (ex. "Why did you _____?", "Are you ___ with me?") in two out of four opportunities to help reduce anxiety by improving communication.

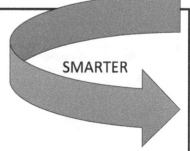

SMARTER

Conclusion

Seems easy, huh?! It is one thing to read and understand the clinical reasoning process, but another to apply it. With that in mind, we encourage you to begin your practice of the goal-writing skillset!

What follows is a number of case studies divided by educational and medical settings. Please use Appendix 4, the clinical reasoning framework, to walk through each step in the process. If you feel stuck, we encourage you to reference the supplementary materials and videos that demonstrate the goal-writing process between adult and pediatric patients, student clinicians, and clinical supervisors. Keep in mind that practicing this framework is the best way to acquire this essential skillset.

Now, let's enjoy some brownies!

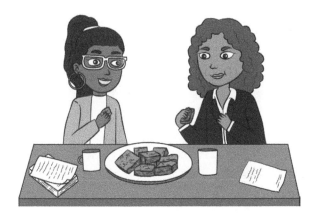

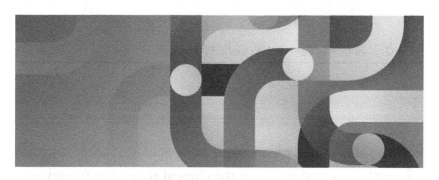

4 Case Studies for Practice

Introduction

This chapter includes 12 case studies that allow you to practice goal writing skills using the clinical reasoning framework. These case studies are intended as a representative sample of commonly encountered patient diagnoses and life circumstances. The first four cases describe adult neurogenic, the next four describe pediatric medical, and the final four describe educational cases. There is no requirement to work in order; rather, choose what seems most relevant to your professional development.

Adult Medical

Dysphagia: Julia

Who Are They?

Medical Information. Julia is a 63-year-old right-handed woman who sustained a brainstem stroke five months prior. She has a medical history of high blood pressure, cholesterolemia, and atrial fibrillation, which for years were left unmanaged due to inadequate health insurance. According to her family, the morning of her stroke, Julia fell out of bed and was unable to speak or swallow. She received PT, OT, and SLP services in the hospital while social workers submitted necessary documentation to establish Medicaid coverage. After seven weeks, she was released to a skilled nursing facility (SNF) where she has resided for eight months. According to physical therapy reports, despite right upper and lower extremity hemiparesis, she can walk safely with the use of a walker. Based on patient request, she is being referred for swallowing treatment.

Educational Information and Language Experience. Julia received a high-school diploma, but her medical history indicates that she has struggled with dyslexia throughout her life. Julia's primary language is English. According to her sister, their father and his side of the family is Portuguese speaking, so the siblings understand Portuguese; however, Julia and her immediate family communicate in English at home and in the community.

What Is Their Current Communication and Swallowing Status?

Diagnostic Assessments. Julia was administered a modified barium swallow study (MBSS) while she was in the hospital. During the exam, she exhibited a delayed swallowing reflex and episodic aspiration based on consistency. Trace aspiration was observed with thin- and nectar-thick liquids followed by a weak cough. The patient managed honey-thick liquids and puree aside from moderate residue in the pyriform sinuses that cleared with repeated swallows and chin tuck posture. A recent evaluation by ENT diagnosed her with hemiparesis of the left vocal folds. During a bedside exam at the skilled nursing facility (SNF), Julia demonstrated impaired oral preparation with trials of soft solids but no signs of aspiration with trials of liquids. She continues to be on a diet of honey-thick liquids and puree.

In addition to swallowing deficits, Julia performed in the moderately impaired range on a motor speech protocol. Noted deficits included impaired vocal quality characterized by breathiness, restricted vocal range, and low volume, and moderately impaired articulatory precision due to reduced lingual strength and range of motion. She performed in the normal range on the Cognitive-Linguistic Quick Test (CLQT; Helm-Estabrooks et al., 2001) with no difficulties noted in language or cognition.

Diagnostic Decisions. Julia presents with moderate oral-pharyngeal dysphagia and mixed flaccid-spastic dysarthria. Her current diet is highly restrictive for safety reasons.

What Is Important to Them?

Interests/Life Events. Before her stroke, Julia worked as an assembler at a dry-cleaning business. Her sister reported that she had worked at that business for over 25 years and was considering retiring once she was eligible for Medicare. In her free time, Julia enjoyed playing competitive pool and in fact used to travel to competitions where she would win money. In recent years, she started playing poker in competitive tournaments as well.

Julia has been divorced for 15 years. She has two children in their 40s whom she rarely sees, although in the past she enjoyed FaceTiming with her grandchildren during holidays. Her sister visits two to three times per week.

Environment. Because of her inability to live independently due to mobility limitations, Julia will be staying at the SNF for the foreseeable future. She has a roommate, but the two do not interact. Julia rarely engages with any other residents or the staff. She sits alone or withdrawn from conversations during meals, and she stays in her room watching television most of the day.

Patient and Family Priorities. Julia reported to her sister that she hates honey-thick liquids and pureed foods. Her sister wants Julia to enjoy her new home as much as possible, but she reports feeling helpless about the situation.

Aphasia: Elisabeth

Who Are They?

Medical Information. Elisabeth is a 68-year-old woman who suffered a left MCA infarct two years ago. Imaging results reveal a large left inferior frontal lesion affecting both the pars triangularis and pars orbicularis. In addition to language deficits, Elisabeth presents with decorticate posturing that impacts her gait and use of her right arm. After the stroke, she received inpatient rehabilitation for six weeks and was then discharged home. Elisabeth attended outpatient physical and speech therapies for five weeks, but she chose to discontinue services because of her inability to communicate effectively with the therapists. Elisabeth's daughter wants her mother to try speech therapy again, because she reportedly seems depressed.

Educational Information and Language Experience. Elisabeth was educated in Germany and earned the equivalent of a bachelor's degree in business. She is a German-English bilingual speaker who is dominant in German. German is her preferred language when she is at home and in social situations with peers and family. In school, Elizabeth achieved moderate English proficiency, but she did not use the language again until arriving in the United States two and a half years ago to help raise her grandchildren. According to her daughter's responses on the Language Experience and Proficiency Questionnaire (LEAP; Marian et al., 2007), Elisabeth is exposed to English 20% of the time, specifically when she accompanies her family to restaurants or the grocery store or when the family is watching television.

What Is Their Current Communication and Swallowing Status?

Diagnostic Assessments. The rehabilitation facility does not have a German-speaking speech-language pathologist, but an interpreter was hired to assist in administering assessments. Elisabeth was given the German version of the Bilingual Aphasia Test (BAT; Paradis & Libben, 1987) and the screener in English. In German, Elisabeth showed significant difficulties in expressive language characterized predominantly by nouns with few verbs, limited bound grammatical morphemes and some apraxic errors such as sound substitutions and cluster reductions. Scores indicated functional receptive language, although she did struggle with semi-complex commands and complex syntactic structures. In English, Elisabeth's spontaneous language consisted of only single-word utterances (all nouns) and she was limited in naming abilities. Her receptive language in English was functional for one-step commands and simple syntactic constructions.

Diagnostic Decisions. Elisabeth presents with functional comprehension, moderate to severe expressive language deficits, and mild apraxia of speech in German, her primary language; she demonstrates similar patterns of deficits in her non-dominant language of English.

What Is Important to Them?

Environment. Elisabeth suffered her stroke soon after arriving in the United States to care for her grandchildren. Although the plan had been for her to assist in the care of the new baby and 3-year-old while her daughter and son-in-law were at work, the parents had to hire a nanny to take over. Since being discharged from rehabilitation, Elisabeth rarely leaves the family home and never on her own. She communicates with her daughter and grandchildren in German, and has brief interactions with her son-in-law in English. She does not attempt to communicate with unfamiliar speakers but lets her daughter speak on her behalf.

Interests/Life Events. Elisabeth was a chef and restaurant owner in a small, northern German town. When the opportunity arose, she happily sold the restaurant and made the decision to focus on family and hobbies. Elisabeth lost her husband in a motor vehicle accident 15 years ago around the same time that her only child got married and moved to the United States. In addition to culinary arts, Elisabeth loves singing and opera.

Patient and Family Priorities. According to her daughter, Elisabeth seems depressed. Not only is she unable to independently care for her grandchildren, but she is scared to attempt to communicate with unfamiliar conversation partners because of her English language skills and aphasia. Elisabeth's goal is to "speak better."

Traumatic Brain Injury: Samuel

Who Are They?

Medical Information. Samuel, a 38-year-old individual who identifies as male (with preferred pronouns they/them), was involved in a motor vehicle accident 9 months prior. They experienced a severe coup-contrecoup injury, which affected prefrontal and occipital-parietal cortices. In the hospital, Samuel underwent a craniectomy to reduce edema and relieve intracranial pressure. They were in a coma for 3 weeks. Once they reached a Ranchos level III (Flannery, 1993; localized response: responds to stimuli specifically and inconsistently with delay;

follows simple commands for motor actions), they were discharged to an inpatient rehabilitation facility where they stayed for 8 weeks. From there, Samuel attended a transitional rehabilitation program for 4 weeks. According to therapy notes from the second program, Samuel made significant progress and was deemed safe to go home as long as the family provided sufficient support specifically for safety.

Educational Information and Language Experience. Samuel completed an associate's degree in web design. Prior to the accident, they were working toward a bachelor's degree in cybersecurity. They are a monolingual English speaker.

What Is Their Current Communication and Swallowing Status?

Diagnostic Assessments. Samuel's performance on the Functional Assessment of Verbal Reasoning and Executive Strategies (FAVRES; Macdonald, 2005) showed significant difficulties with reasoning (standard score of 79, 5th percentile) including weighing facts, eliminating irrelevant information, and cognitive flexibility. Though able to read short texts, they were disorganized in their approach to visual information (scanning quickly, failing to recheck information, etc.). Their spontaneous speech sample showed intact microstructure (i.e., grammatical components, lexical diversity), but deficits in story grammar organization and topic maintenance. Samuel needed frequent breaks throughout the evaluation and was highly distracted by noise in the hallway. Other qualitative observations included impaired pragmatics such as nervous laughter and socially inappropriate behavior (e.g., picking their nose during the evaluation).

Diagnostic Decisions. Samuel presents with moderately impaired cognitive-communication characterized by deficits in higher-level executive functions (inhibitory control, organization and planning), sustained attention, pragmatic language and self-awareness. Language expression and comprehension are intact.

What Is Important to Them?

Environment. Samuel is married with three school-aged children. During the day, Samuel stays with their grandmother who is retired and primarily stays at home. Samuel's grandmother dotes on her grandchild by cooking them meals and catering to their needs. The television is kept at a loud volume for most of the day while Samuel plays games on their phone and surfs internet travel sites. In the evenings and on weekends, Samuel continues these same activities while their wife, Adriana, and children run errands, attend sports practices and birthday parties, and go to church functions. According to Adriana, Samuel is detached from the family; the children do not interact with their father who rarely initiates conversation with them. Adriana disclosed that she is in counseling to address feelings of hopelessness with her home life.

Interests/Life Events. Prior to the accident, Samuel was a highly driven individual with a number of interests. They worked full-time as a web designer at a private consulting firm and attended school in the evenings. Samuel shared in the evaluation that they would love to continue pursuing their associate's degree, but coursework was currently impossible because the doctor insisted that their driver's license be suspended. Samuel was also a trumpet player in a jazz band that performed at local clubs once a month (they have not picked up an instrument since the accident). Samuel used to love traveling as well. Although they had not traveled overseas in many years, the family used to explore one to two national parks per year.

Patient and Family Priorities. Samuel stated that their primary goal is to drive again. Being able to drive would enable them to return to school and work and contribute to home life by going grocery shopping and paying bills. They acknowledged that their wife needs help. As Adriana listened to her husband's response, she quietly shook her head and stated, "But they can't even get ready without help in the morning." Adriana wants her spouse to participate in the family and "lead a productive life, whatever that looks like."

Parkinson's Disease: Tomas

Who Are They?

Medical Information. Tomas is a 57-year-old man who went to his primary care physician at his spouse's insistence due to complaints of tremor in his hands and others' reports of his worsening "mumbling." He was referred to neurology, where he received a diagnosis of Parkinson's disease. Three months ago he began taking Levadopa, which reportedly improved his physical symptoms, but not his intelligibility. His medical history is otherwise unremarkable.

Educational Information and Language Experience. Tomas has a master's degree in business administration and is proficient in French, Spanish, and Arabic. Because his mother was in the U.S. State Department, Tomas attended international schools in Paris and Morocco. He returned to the United States for college, which included one year on a study abroad program in Madrid. He reports speaking English 90% of the time; the other languages he uses at work with business clients. English is his preferred language when he is at home with his family.

What Is Their Current Communication and Swallowing Status?

Diagnostic Assessments. The neurologist referred Tomas for a speech/voice evaluation (swallowing is not a concern at this time). An oral-motor exam revealed symmetrical function but mildly reduced range of motion of the articulators and facial muscles. Results from the Sentence Intelligibility Test (Yorkston et al., 1996), showed mildly impaired intelligibility for single words, but moderate impairments at the sentence level. Tomas's speech and vocal production was remarkable for increased rate (up to 180 words per minute), reduced articulatory precision, mild breathiness, and low intensity due to reduced respiratory support. Tomas scored in the mild-moderate range on the 9-item Voice Handicap Index (Nawka et al., 2009), indicating that he perceives that his declining speech and voice abilities are impacting his quality of life at home and at work.

Diagnostic Decisions. Tomas presents with mild-moderate hypokinetic dysarthria that includes the motor speech subsystems of respiration, phonation, and articulation.

What Is Important to Them?

Environment. Tomas works for a venture capital firm and he intends to continue working for as long as possible. He is a self-disclosed workaholic who works 60-hour weeks and travels up to 10 days per month. His days are filled with conference calls, meetings on Zoom, and live presentations in large conference rooms. Tomas has been married to his second wife, Nicole, for eight years and they have a 4- and 6-year-old. He also has two children from his first marriagem whom he typically sees twice a year during their university breaks. Nicole reports that her husband is involved in family life on weekends including participating in some birthday parties and playdates. The couple enjoys dinners and other social events with friends at least twice a month.

Interests/Life Events. With his demanding work and family life, Tomas has little time for hobbies. He used to belong to an adult choir but chose to step away because of the time commitment, although he reported that he would love to return in the future. Tomas also shared that he has a secret passion for art history, his minor in college. Tomas enjoys reading to his young children in the evenings when he is not working or out of town.

Patient and Family Priorities. Tomas stated that he is tired of being told by his wife and children to talk louder. He acknowledged feeling embarrassed when asked to use a microphone during presentations at work, and he would love to be able to project his voice like he used to. Nicole has noticed a decrease in their ability to communicate as a couple, and she finds herself needing to clarify and/or rephrase what her husband is trying to say in social contexts.

Pediatric Medical

Fluency: Roshan

Who Are They?

Medical Information. Roshan is a 14-year-old male who was diagnosed with stuttering at the age of 4 years old. He has a positive family history of stuttering as his paternal grandfather stuttered. Roshan received speech therapy from the age of 4 to

7 years old in an outpatient setting. His language and speech skills were within normal limits and the focus of outpatient therapy for Roshan was communication and self-advocacy. His parents stopped sending him to therapy as Roshan was getting busy with after-school activities and they perceived that he was communicating effectively and was happy. Roshan was reported to have a history of multiple ear infections between the ages of 2 and 4. He also wears corrective lenses.

Educational Information and Language Experience. Roshan is currently in the 8th grade at a local middle school and is a monolingual English speaker. Academically, he is doing well overall with A and B grades in his classes; however, he struggled to get a B in ceramics. Roshan excels in math, is on the chess team, and in the marching band. His dream is to become a drum major in high school. This year, he is required to read, give oral presentations, and answer questions out loud during class for a participation grade. He reported to his parents that he feels a lot of pressure in his classes and that he stutters a lot more and is having a difficult time managing the pressure of his required speaking and his stuttering at the same time. During classes when he raises his hand and is called on, he reports that he stutters almost every time and that he is getting increasingly negative reactions from his classmates about his stuttering. He recently stopped raising his hand in class and refused to give a required oral presentation resulting in the teacher contacting his parents about compliance in class.

What Is Their Current Communication and Swallowing Status?

Diagnostic Assessments. At Roshan's request, his parents brought him into an outpatient setting for therapy in the hope of helping him better manage his stuttering in school. Based on the Stuttering Severity Instrument-4 (SSI-4; Riley & Bakker, 2009), Roshan's stuttering was in the moderate range with the presence of secondary characteristics (e.g., eye blinks, hand tapping) and stuttering-like disfluencies during speaking and reading tasks. Based on his responses on the Overall Assessment of the Speaker's Experience of Stuttering for Teens (OASES-T; Yaruss & Quesal, 2016), Roshan exhibited a moderate to severe impact rating on his quality of life as further justification for therapy.

Diagnostic Decisions. Roshan exhibits stuttering with a moderate severity rating and a moderate to severe impact on his quality of life.

What Is Important to Them?

Environment. Roshan feels significant pressures at school due to increased required speaking demands and the recent negative reactions from peers. He feels that he communicates more effectively in small groups of close peers and at home. He tends to stutter less when he is gaming with friends using his headset to communicate. Additionally, he is comfortable in the band hall with his fellow bandmates and with select chess team members. At home, his fluency waxes and wanes depending on how tired he is. His parents disclosed he feels additional stress when talking to girls in his class and spends a lot of time on social media.

Patient and Family Priorities. Roshan expressed wanting to practice strategies for communicating more fluently during required classroom-type tasks. He also stated wanting to develop a comeback to use in response to negative comments or reactions about his stuttering. His parents want him to feel confident and included, but do not want to receive additional phone calls from the school.

Speech Sound Disorder: Jeremiah

Who Are They?

Medical Information. Jeremiah is a 4-year, 9-month-old male referred for an initial speech-language evaluation by his pediatrician during his three-year checkup. The family has not been able to obtain an evaluation until now. Pregnancy and birth were reported to be unremarkable and no history of allergies or medications were reported. He reportedly had difficulty latching and was bottle fed. His hearing was screened at the time of the evaluation and passed bilaterally.

Developmental Information. Per parent report, Jeremiah walked at 14 months of age and was toilet trained at 23 months. He spoke his first words at 16 months of age and combined two-word utterances at 20 months. He is reported to follow multi-step commands and demonstrates age-appropriate comprehension. His mother reported that she is only able to understand 50% of his utterances. His older brother and sister were reportedly more successful at understanding his speech. Per parent report, Jeremiah is unaware of his speech sound errors and only becomes frustrated when asked to repeat an utterance multiple times. Jeremiah prefers toys with moving parts and lights.

Educational Information and Language Experience. Currently, Jeremiah attends a preschool program three times per week at the neighborhood church. He is one of ten children of similar age who participate in this program. His teacher reported that Jeremiah engages actively with his peers and does not seem to be phased or aware when his peers do not understand him. However, with teachers, they observed behaviors of frustration as demonstrated by sighs, disengagement, and refusing to eat when his preferred choices are not understood (i.e., when communicating snack preference). His mid-year report indicated that Jeremiah can identify letters based upon their sounds but is unable to consistently produce letter sounds. Jeremiah and his family are monolingual English speakers. There is minimal exposure to other languages in his immediate environment.

What Is Their Current Communication and Swallowing Status?

Diagnostic Assessments. A battery of speech and language assessments were administered which included the Auditory Comprehension subtest of the Preschool Language Scale–5th Edition (PLS-5; Zimmerman et al., 2011), Goldman-Fristoe Test of Articulation–3rd Edition (GTFA-3; Goldman & Fristoe, 2015), a hearing screening, oral peripheral examination, and dynamic assessment. Age-appropriate comprehension was noted on the PLS-5. Jeremiah obtained a standard score of 46 on the Sounds-In-Words subtest of the GFTA-3. Based upon his productions, the Khan-Lewis Phonological Analysis-Third Edition (KLPA-3; Khan & Lewis, 2015) was completed and a high occurrence of the following processes were noted: stopping of fricatives and affricates, final consonant deletion, gliding of liquids, vowelization, and palatal fronting. During a dynamic assessment, sound approximation elicitation methods were used to transition productions from /t/ to /s/. Jeremiah required verbal prompting for tensing lingual muscles when producing /t/ and visual cues to elongate the production of /ts/ without the presence of lateral airflow. Through direct modeling, instructional prompts, and multiple trials, Jeremiah displayed stimulability for the production of /s/ in isolation; however, he was unable to maintain the production across trials and/or time. Discoordination and misarticulations were noted within his sequential and variable diadochokinetic rates. Decreased rate of speech improved production and accuracy.

Diagnostic Decisions. Jeremiah was diagnosed with a severe phonological processing disorder with respect to his chronological age. He demonstrates speech sound production errors that are considered developmentally significant and impact his expressive language abilities. These errors severely affect Jeremiah's overall intelligibility during communicative interactions particularly with unfamiliar listeners.

What Is Important to Them?

Environment. Jeremiah currently lives at home with his father, mother, older brother, and older sister. Both sets of grandparents and several cousins live in the area and are active participants in his life.

Interests/Life Events. The family is active in their church in which Jeremiah attends a Sunday school class and participates in weekly children's programming. His parents report that Jeremiah enjoys playing team sports including soccer and t-ball. He loves sorting and organizing objects, but has a particular affinity for sorting recyclables.

Patient and Family Priorities. Jeremiah's parents expressed concern with the emergence of frustration; particularly, at his school. They are worried that his speech will impact his success in kindergarten both socially and academically.

Feeding and Swallowing: Grady

Who Are They?

Medical Information. Grady is a 3-year-old child who presented with severe food refusal and oral aversion. He prefers drinking liquids rather than eating solid foods; however, he has an affinity for orange-colored foods. His mother reported a normal pregnancy and delivery. There is no reported history of allergies. Per parent report, there is no history or overt signs of gastrointestinal issues. He was reported to have infrequent bouts of constipation, which were resolved with over-the-counter medication. He was reported to be growing well but is on the lower end of weight and height. His vision and hearing were reportedly not assessed since birth; however, no concerns were expressed by the mother.

Developmental Information. Grady was reported to meet all gross motor milestones to date. Difficulty with the use of a spoon and fork were noted. He is not currently toilet trained. His mother expressed concern about communication skills; however, her primary concern was his feeding skills. Grady was reported to eat limited volumes of solid foods and prefers drinking (large volumes) over eating.

Educational Information and Language Experience. Grady attends daycare from 7:00 am to 6:00 pm daily, Monday through Friday. Grady and his family are monolingual English speakers.

What Is Their Current Communication and Swallowing Status?

Diagnostic Assessments. Grady was referred for a feeding evaluation at an outpatient pediatric rehabilitation center. Grady was reported to have limited acceptance of fruit, meats, and grains. He will not consume any vegetables and was reported to graze on foods throughout the day. During the assessment, there were no observable signs or symptoms of swallowing difficulty. According to a parent-reported food diary from the previous day, food intake involved the following:

- Breakfast: He was offered oatmeal and Cheerios but refused—he drank 4 ounces of Pediasure mixed with whole milk (1:1 ratio).
- Snack: He was offered breakfast at daycare and took two bites.
- Lunch: At daycare refused solids and consumed all liquid provided. At home he ate a strawberry Go-gurt yogurt and two bites of a granola bar.
- Snack: His daycare teacher offered solids of raisins and cheese, but he only took two bites of raisins and refused the cheese; he drank water.
- Dinner: He refused the family meal and then was given two Danimals yogurts.

Grady was reported to consume 27 ounces of whole milk per day, 16 ounces of Pediasure per day, three to four ounces of juice per day, and eight ounces of water per day. During the evaluation, Grady was observed self-feeding Goldfish using a vertical chewing pattern for five to seven bites with intermittent sucking. Sucking increased with manipulation of a pretzel stick. He was offered oatmeal from home and presented with severe refusal behaviors of turning away and crying.

Diagnostic Decisions. Grady presents with a severe feeding disorder characterized by limited oral intake of solid foods and decreased diversity in his diet.

What Is Important to Them?

Environment. Grady lives at home with his parents and two sisters, ages one and a half and five years of age. He does not participate in after-school activities such as soccer and has limited time away from his parents due to his feeding restrictions and behaviors. He was reported to only play independently in group settings. Parents reported attempting t-ball last year; however, Grady refused to participate after the first game. His mother suspected this was due to not enjoying the snacks presented after the game. He was reported to have a meltdown when another mom insisted that he take a slice of pizza.

Interests/Life Events. Grady loves toy cars, pretend play, and the Cars movie.

Patient and Family Priorities. Grady's parents would love for him to participate in meals at both daycare and at home without consistent refusal. They are frustrated by his dependence on specific foods that affect his ability to participate in social interactions. His behaviors seem to be increasing which is also an area of concern.

Craniofacial Syndrome: Sloane

Who Are They?

Medical Information. Sloane is a 23-month-old child with a history of cleft palate. Palate repair was completed around approximately 12 months of age. Sloane has been followed by a cleft palate team since birth and will meet with the team on an annual basis post-palate repair. Her history is significant for supplemental feedings through g-tube, oral feeding difficulties, and dysphagia of thin liquids. Currently, Sloane meets all nutrition and hydration needs by mouth with no concern. Sloane had bilateral ear tubes placed by the ENT at the time of the cleft-palate repair because of a history of bilateral conductive hearing loss. Currently, Sloane presents with flat tympanograms/open tubes and normal sound-field testing.

Developmental Information. Sloane previously qualified for early childhood intervention (ECI) services for physical, occupational, and feeding therapy within the home. She has mastered her goals for physical and feeding therapy and continues to receive ECI services one time per month for occupational therapy. To date, speech therapy services were reported to primarily focus on feeding skills due to decreased oral intake and body weight. Speech therapy for communication skills was recommended but had not started.

Educational Information and Language Experience. Sloane stays home with a caregiver during the day who reads books and watches daytime television at loud volume. Sloane, her caregiver, and her parents are monolingual English speakers.

What Is Their Current Communication and Swallowing Status?

Diagnostic Assessments. Her cleft palate team referred her for a more in-depth speech and language evaluation after her last visit. Prior to the evaluation, Sloane had completed occupational and speech therapy sessions within her home so she was low energy and fell asleep at the end of the assessment. Standardized assessment was attempted and not completed due to lack of participation and tolerance of activities. The PLS-5 (Zimmerman et al., 2011) was completed using criterion-referenced methods. Her parents reported that Sloane is vocal throughout the day and enjoys social play. She was reported to consistently use the phoneme /m/ and attempt to verbalize "mama." According to her mother, she responds to her name, understands routine phrase words like "nigh nigh" and "bye bye," and recognizes words for common items.

Diagnostic Decisions. Sloane presents with a severe speech and language delay characterized by decreased expressive language and a restricted phonemic inventory.

What Is Important to Them?

Environment. Sloane lives at home with her parents and an older brother who is 10 years old. They have limited family support. Both parents work outside the home to help with the cost of medical care for Sloane.

Interests/Life Events. Sloane is reported to have limited interaction with same-age peers. Her parents work opposing work schedules. Her parents felt that it was important to limit Sloane's exposure to germs to avoid delays in care and the need for additional days off of work. She enjoys watching Bluey and Cocomelon. Her favorite toys are her play kitchen and baby doll, Sally.

Patient and Family Priorities. Now that Sloane's feeding skills have improved and her palate repair was successful, her parents are excited to focus on other areas of her development and to potentially increase her socialization with same-age peers such as play dates with neighborhood children.

Education

Developmental Language Disorder— School Age: Carla

Who Are They?

Developmental Information. Carla is a 5-year-old-girl who lives with her grandparents. According to her grandmother,

Carla is physically healthy, and she met all gross motor developmental milestones (crawling and walking). Her grandmother reported that Carla did not start talking until she was 3 years old in contrast with Carla's two older sisters who started talking at much younger ages. In the home, Carla relies on her sisters for guidance in activities and communicates in short phrases in both English and Spanish. Carla had a tonsillectomy and adenoidectomy at the age of 3. She reportedly forgets to manage her saliva when excited.

Educational Information and Language Experience. Carla attends a local elementary school where she is in a Spanish-English bilingual kindergarten classroom. She receives 50% instruction in each language. Her teacher recently raised concerns that Carla seems "lost" during the day and has a hard time following routines such as circle time and participating in small group center activities. Carla does not follow directions well in either language and seems to rely on copying what other children are doing (e.g., getting up to stand in line only after seeing friends do so). During small group time, Carla rarely speaks to the other children except for a few words in English or Spanish and she prefers to play by herself or with one other friend in the classroom. The teacher reported that Carla primarily communicates in short phrases such as "want some snack," "don't see mine friend," and "*quiero casa abuela*/ I want house grandma."

During reading groups, Carla is reportedly not making sufficient progress with letter identification in English or Spanish. She knows some short sight words in each language but she struggles with phonological awareness and writing letters. She can count to 50 in English with some assistance although this skill is not developed in Spanish. In addition to concerns with overall communication in both languages, Carla's teacher is worried about her reading readiness and functional literacy skills particularly because it is nearly the end of the Fall term.

What Is Their Current Communication and Swallowing Status?

Diagnostic Assessments. Carla scored two standard deviations below the mean on administered subtests of the Bilingual English Spanish Assessment (BESA; Peña et al., 2018). Overall, her scores in English and Spanish were comparable; she scored higher on the semantics subtests than on the morphosyntax subtests in both languages. Scores on the semantics subtests were within one standard deviation from the mean (low average range). On the English morphosyntax subtest, she exhibited difficulties with the past tense morpheme (-ed) and prepositions (e.g., beside). In Spanish, she exhibited difficulties with direct object clitics (*lo/los, la/las*) and relative clauses (*la mama recoge el niño que lleva puesto el suéter azul*/the mom picks up the boy who is wearing a blue sweater). In both languages she had difficulty answering "where" and "why" questions and also comprehension questions about a short narrative. Language sample data from narrative retells corroborated the standardized testing. Carla produced more ungrammatical than grammatical sentences in both English and Spanish, with lower than average mean length of utterance (MLU) in both languages compared to her bilingual same-age peers. Both grandparents and teachers exhibited concerns about her language skills in English and Spanish through guardian/teacher interviews. Dynamic assessment trials in both languages for grammatical items she missed in testing yielded high clinician effort and minimal change, which is indicative of a language disorder.

Diagnostic Decisions. Carla presents with a moderate developmental language disorder in English and Spanish characterized by difficulties with expressive and receptive language in both verbal and written modalities.

What Is Important to Them?

Environment and Interests/Life Events. In the home setting, Carla relies on her older siblings to "talk" for her. She communicates in short sentences in both languages. Her communication attempts occur primarily when she needs or wants something not in her reach. When she is frustrated at home, she cries or shuts down. Carla's grandmother describes her as a shy, reserved child who seems to prefer time by herself and playing games on her tablet. She enjoys playing Dance Dance Revolution on her Nintendo Switch. She also loves to look at books about cats with her grandmother. At school during small reading groups, Carla has recently started to pick at her cuticles until they bleed.

Patient and Family Priorities. As a priority, Carla's grandparents would like to see improvements in her literacy skills; they are concerned she will fall further behind her peers in reading. They would also like for Carla to communicate in longer sentences so that they understand what she needs the first time she asks for something.

Developmental Language Disorder— Early Childhood: Katelynn

Who Are They?

Medical Information. Katelynn is a 3-year, 2-month-old female who was referred for an initial speech-language evaluation by her pediatrician during a recent visit where she was diagnosed with otitis media. Dr. Torres expressed concerns about Katelynn's language development. Due to financial restraints, Katelynn's parents requested a speech and language evaluation within her local elementary school. Katelynn was born at 37 weeks and experienced neonatal jaundice. Her mother reported difficulty with breastfeeding due to Katelynn having a tongue tie; however, no additional feeding difficulties have been reported. Katelynn has a frequent history of otitis media over the last 9 months which has been resolved through the use of antibiotics.

Developmental Information. Per parent report, Katelynn's gross and fine motor milestones were all met within age-expected ranges. She is currently toilet trained. Katelynn's parents expressed concerns due to her limited vocabulary and lack of use of two-word utterances at home and within community inter-actions. At 18 months of age, Katelynn was evaluated through Early Childhood Intervention (ECI). Her parents reported that Katelynn performed within the expected age range and did not qualify for intervention at that time.

Educational Information and Language Experience. Cur-rently, Katelynn attends a preschool program twice weekly for four hours. Her parents reported that she interacts and plays well with her peers; however, her teachers have noted a difference in her use of language compared to same-age peers. Katelynn is a monolingual English speaker with no exposure to any other languages at home or within the community.

What Is Their Current Communication and Swallowing Status?

Diagnostic Assessments. Katelynn was administered the PLS-5 (Zimmerman et al., 2011). Her auditory comprehension score was 78 with a percentile rank of 12%. Her expressive com-munication standardized score was 76 with a percentile rank of 10%. Difficulties with understanding pronouns and quantitative concepts were noted. She demonstrated joint attention, initiated turn-taking and social routines, and used gestures and vocalizations to request objects. Overall, Katelynn was observed using more gestures and non-words to communicate. The use of two-word utterances was not observed and was unable to be elicited.

Her parents completed the criterion-referenced assessment of the Receptive-Expressive Emergent Language Test–4th Edition (REEL-4; Brown et al., 2020). A standard score of 82 was obtained on the receptive language subtest, and a standard score of 84 was obtained on the expressive language subtest. The overall language ability standard score was reported to be 83.

During a functional play and language sample, Katelynn was observed to use single-scheme combinations and multi-scheme combinations during play. She was observed to manipulate the physical properties of objects and showed joint attention during play activities. Currently, Katelynn was reported using approximately 75 to 100 words consisting primarily of nouns. She utilizes one-word utterances with the addition of pointing and effectively communicates with familiar partners in familiar environments. Her parents report that unfamiliar listeners often have difficulty understanding her speech, and she is hesitant to interact with strangers. She is reported to be able to follow simple and contextual one-step commands at home.

Diagnostic Decisions. Based upon standardized scores, criterion-referenced assessment, parent report, and functional observation, Katelynn presents with a mild-moderate expressive language delay.

What Is Important to Them?

Environment. Katelynn is an only child who lives at home with her parents. Her grandmother provides care for her during the day a few days per week. She has a hamster named George and a bunny named Fluffy.

Interests/Life Events. She actively participates in gymnastics and Kindermusik with same-age peers. In these activities, her mother reported frequently needing to provide redirection. She would also request the bathroom when she disliked specific activities. Her favorite show is Bluey, and she enjoys coloring and riding her scooter with neighborhood children.

Patient and Family Priorities. Increased use of multiword utterances and the ability to use language in cooperative play are high priorities for Katelynn's parents. They would love for her to be an active participant in her social activities.

Speech Sound Disorder: Mei Ling

Who Are They?

Medical Information. Mei Ling is a 5-year-old Mandarin–English bilingual female. Mei Ling has a significant history of otitis media. She had recurrent ear infections starting at 18 months through the age of two and a half years old. She was evaluated by an ENT and received pressure equalization (PE) tubes at age two and a half years old. She received a second set of PE tubes at the age of three. Mei Ling was diagnosed with ADHD at four years of age. Her parents describe her as "always on the go" with a fleeting attention span. Her parents reported a positive family history of speech and language disorders on her father's side including a cousin with a speech disorder and an uncle with a developmental language disorder.

Developmental Information. Mei Ling met fine and gross motor milestones within the average range. She was referred to a speech-language pathologist at the age of three years old due to concerns from her pediatrician that despite the improvement in communication since having PE tubes placed, she was still mostly unintelligible to unfamiliar listeners in English and Mandarin. She received speech therapy for articulation in English and Mandarin from the age of three to four and a half years old and then was discharged from home health speech therapy due to meeting goals for functional communication in the home.

Educational Information and Language Experience. Mei Ling attends kindergarten in an English-only classroom. The teacher is concerned as Mei Ling struggles with socialization and is having trouble making friends. Her teacher reports that peers make quizzical faces at Mei Ling or ask "what did you say?" when she speaks. She is also struggling with social communication and respecting others' social boundaries. Her teacher describes when Mei Ling approaches friends to play, she will take items from other students' hands to take her turn first. Despite verbal and nonverbal cues from her peers, she plays "rough" and does not observe personal space boundaries. During small group intervention the teacher has significant difficulties understanding what Mei Ling is saying, and she has recently noticed that Mei Ling is crying during class and shutting down. Mei Ling does not like when she is asked to repeat herself and is becoming increasingly frustrated when this occurs. Her teacher is concerned that her unintelligible speech and challenging social skills are impeding Mei Ling's ability to participate in daily learning activities.

Mei Ling resides in a bilingual English- and Mandarin-speaking home. Her parents speak both Mandarin and English to her while her grandparents only speak and understand Mandarin. A language history questionnaire revealed that Mei Ling is exposed to and uses Mandarin 40% and English 60% of the time. Mei Ling code-switches (uses words from one language in another language) when she is speaking in the home. Mei Ling only uses English at school.

What Is Their Current Communication and Swallowing Status?

Diagnostic Assessments. As part of the multi-tiered system of support (MTSS) process, Mei Ling received a formal speech and language evaluation. She scored within the average range on the Clinical Evaluation of Language Fundamentals Preschool language screening test (CELF Preschool-3 Screening Test; Wiig et al., 2020). The speech-language pathologists administered the Goldman-Fristoe Test of Articulation–3rd Edition (GFTA-3; Goldman & Fristoe, 2015) in English and then cross-referenced any articulation or phonological error patterns to those found in Mandarin. She scored more than one standard deviation below the mean on the GFTA-3. After cross-referencing the error patterns, the clinician found that Mei Ling exhibited consistent errors on 5 different overlapping sounds present in both English and Mandarin (/s/, /k/, /t/, /m/, /f/) and one sound unique to English (/g/). With the help of a Mandarin-speaking interpreter, the clinician probed sounds unique to Mandarin at the word level to see if she exhibited any articulation errors. The SLP found that she produced errors on the following sounds unique to Mandarin (/tʰ/, /kʰ/, aspirated sounds) Mei Ling's intelligibility to an unfamiliar listener was rated at 50% in English and 40% in Mandarin.

Diagnostic Decision. Mei Ling exhibits an articulation disorder in both languages characterized by sound distortions and substitution errors.

What Is Important to Them?

Environment. She is an only child who lives with her parents and grandparents. She attends the neighborhood ballet school and enjoys going to the farmers' market with her family.

Patient and Family Priorities. Mei Ling's parents are concerned about the challenges she experiences with friends. They feel her articulation and social skills are impeding her ability to interact with other children. Her parents would like for Mei Ling to be more understandable.

Developmental Language Disorder— School Age: Daniel

Who Are They?

Developmental Information. Daniel is a 9-year-old-male who lives at home with his mother, father, and older brother. Daniel is in overall good health. His mother reported that he started talking around two and half years old and met other major milestones such as crawling and walking on time. There is a family history of communication disorders: a maternal uncle was diagnosed with autism and a second cousin was recently diagnosed with developmental language disorder (DLD). Daniel's older brother was also diagnosed with DLD and received speech and language services through middle school.

Educational Information and Language Experience. Daniel is in the fourth grade at a local public school in an English-speaking classroom. He has limited exposure to other languages; he and his family are monolingual English speakers. During the last round of teacher conferences, Daniel's teachers raised concerns about his understanding of grade-level oral and written text. His teacher reported that he struggles with word problems in math and does much better when he just works with numbers and equations alone. Further, he struggles with understanding complex sentences and answering questions related to what he has read resulting in low scores on his reading benchmark testing. Daniel's teacher is concerned that he does not understand what he reads and that he will continue to fall further behind his peers. His teacher recently noticed that he is withdrawing from peers and not participating in group activities.

What Is Their Current Communication and Swallowing Status?

Diagnostic Assessments. As part of the multi-tiered system of support (MTSS) process, Daniel was referred for a full speech and language evaluation as he was not making gains in the classroom with the teacher and SLP consulting on strategies to help Daniel such as a buddy to help him when he gets "lost" in activity directions, additional small group intervention time focused on reading multisyllabic words, and increased comprehension checks based on what he has read. He scored more than one standard deviation on the Oral Written Language Scales (OWLS-2, Carrow-Woolfolk, 2011) Oral Expression and Listening Comprehension subtests. He also scored below average on the Gray Oral Reading Test Fifth Edition (GORT-5; Wiederholt & Bryant, 2012). During dynamic assessment, Daniel exhibited low modifiability to structured teaching of areas he struggled with on the OWLS-2 such as understanding relative clauses. During a classroom observation, Daniel refused to read aloud when the teacher encouraged him to take his turn. While in small group time with a math lesson, Daniel turned his head away and looked down when peers were discussing their task instructions. He did not ask for assistance.

Diagnostic Decisions. Based on evaluation results, Daniel exhibits DLD with specific challenges in understanding higher-level complex/abstract language and reading comprehension. He is in need of services as his DLD is impacting his access to the curriculum.

What Is Important to Them?

Environment and Interests/Life Events. Daniel enjoys imaginative play with peers. He wants to take part in socializing with friends on the playground and at lunchtime but is often excluded. When he tries to participate, he often takes longer to respond, so peers assume that he has nothing to say. At home, Daniel's interactions with his brother are more successful because they have learned each other's communication styles. Both brothers are reported to be interested in Roblox and Minecraft.

Patient and Family Priorities. Daniel wants to participate in small group activities in the classroom. His family also expressed that they would like for him to gain confidence in his reading ability and participate in small groups with peers. Daniel's father would like for him to participate in group sports, preferably football.

Conclusion

We hope that these case studies provide sufficient practice of this important skillset. For more support, please access the supplementary content that includes videos of two case studies in which novice clinicians are guided through the clinical reasoning framework to write meaningful goals for their clients.

We wish you luck in your future baking endeavors!

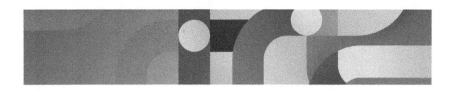

Appendix 1

Factors That Inform Clinical Reasoning

Clinician Factors	Setting Factors	Patient Factors
Clinical experiences	Environmental characteristics	Social-emotional characteristics
Life circumstances	Frequency and duration of services	Personal goals
Personal experiences	Third party demands	Individual performance during assessments
Social-emotional characteristics	Site specific procedures	Medical and rehabilitation history
Cognitive factors related to clinician's own use of logic/ judgment	Practice guidelines & scope of practice relative to training/ equipment available	Abilities and experiences
		Developmental and educational skills

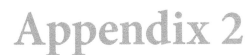

Appendix 2

Cognitive Processes That Inform Clinical Reasoning

Prototypes	"The clinician's background knowledge, domain-specific knowledge, or internal database of characteristics associated with particular diagnoses" *
Logic	The process by which an individual reaches a conclusion
Inductive reasoning (data-driven logic)	The clinician examines the information and draws a conclusion based on the presented facts
Deductive reasoning (hypothesis-driven logic)	The clinician first considers a prototype to solve the problem and then reaches a solution based on the most relevant prototype

*Ginsberg et al., 2016; Harjai & Tiwari, 2009, p. 306

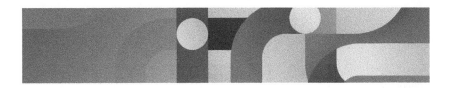

Appendix 3

Data That Inform Clinical Reasoning

Key Question:	Data Type	Description
Who is the patient?	Medical information	Medical diagnoses; comorbidities, medications; allergies; hearing and vision status; maternal health and birth history; feeding/swallowing history; diet restrictions; mobility limitations; significant medical events such as illnesses, injuries, and surgeries; and previous history of therapies.
	Developmental information	The patient's achievement of developmental milestones in areas such as fine motor, gross motor, cognitive skills, and speech and language.
	Educational information	Pediatric patients: The potential functional impact of communication deficits on the ability to function and thrive within a learning environment.
		Adult patients: The patient's level of education to inform literacy and language use, and also vocational or occupational training.
	Language experience	The patient's exposure and use of language(s) and dialects.

continues

continued

Key Question:	Data Type	Description
What is their current communication and swallowing status?	Diagnostic assessments	Performance measures: standardized or criterion-referenced instruments and qualitative measures (language sampling) that assess an area of concern for the patient.
	Diagnostic decisions	The differential diagnostic process in which patient-relevant information is combined with performance measures to form clinical impressions.
What is important to them?	Environment	Communicative settings in which a patient lives and participates.
	Interests / life events	Past, present, and future interests and/or life events that include specific activities or tasks, psychological well-being, and/or academic or social achievements.
	Patient and family priorities	Information and goals of value to the patient and family; there is a direct correlation between the perceived value of therapy services and the inclusion of these priorities in the therapeutic process.

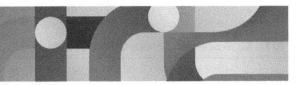

Clinical Reasoning Goal Writing Template

Appendix 4

Clinical Reasoning Goal Writing Template

Clinical Reasoning Goal Writing Template

Goal Planning:

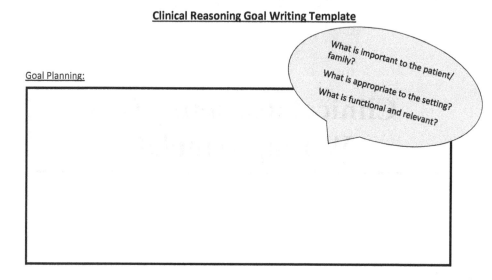

Synthesis:

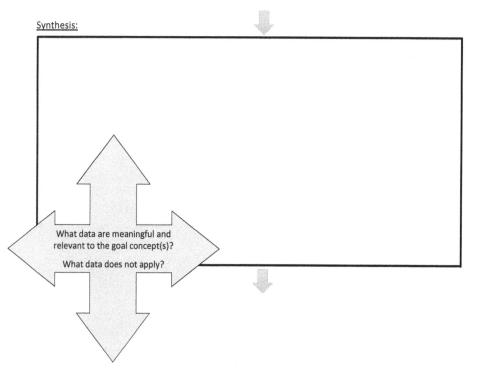

Connection:

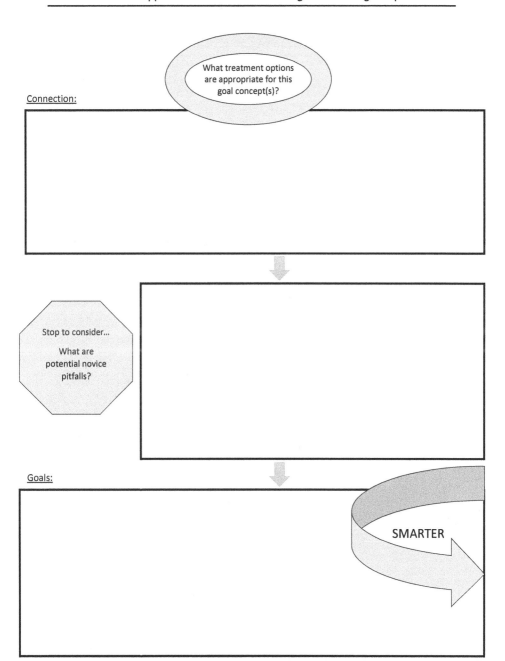

Stop to consider...

What are potential novice pitfalls?

What treatment options are appropriate for this goal concept(s)?

Goals:

SMARTER

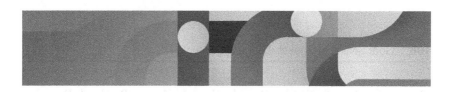

References

Abendroth, K. J., & Whited, J. E. (2021). Motivation, rapport, and resilience: Three pillars of adolescent therapy to shift the focus to adulthood. *Perspectives of the ASHA Special Interest Groups, 6*(5), 1254–1262. https://doi.org/10.1044/2021_persp-20-00289

American Speech-Language-Hearing Association. (n.d.-a). *Fluency disorders.* https://www.asha.org/practice-portal/clinical-topics/fluency-disorders/#collapse_4

American Speech-Language-Hearing Association. (n.d.-b). *Evidence-based practice.* https://www.asha.org/research/ebp/

American Speech-Language-Hearing Association. (n.d.-c). *Person- and family-centered care.* (https://www.asha.org/practice-portal/clinical-topics/aphasia/person-and-family-centered-care/)

Anakin, M., Jouart, M., Timmermans, J., & Pinnock, R. (2020). Student experiences of learning clinical reasoning. *The Clinical Teacher, 17*(1), 52–57. https://doi.org/10.1111/tct.13014

Benfield, A. M., & Johnston, M. V. (2020). Initial development of a measure of evidence-informed professional thinking. *Australian Occupational Therapy Journal, 67*(4), 309–319. https://doi.org/10.1111/1440-1630.12655

Bowen J. L. (2006). Educational strategies to promote clinical diagnostic reasoning. *The New England Journal of Medicine, 355*(21), 2217–2225. https://doi.org/10.1056/NEJMra054782

Brown, V. L., Bzoch, K. R., & League, R. (2020). *Receptive-Expressive Emergent Language Test-4 (REEL-4).* Pro-Ed.

Carrow-Woolfolk, E. (2011). *Oral and Written Language Scales Second Edition (OWLS-II).* WPS.

Centre for Neuro Skills. *Rancho Los Amigos - Revised.* Rancho Los Amigos Revised. (n.d.). https://www.neuroskills.com /education-and-resources/rancho-los-amigos-revised/

Coker, P. (2009). Effects of an experiential learning program on the clinical reasoning and critical thinking skills of occupational therapy students. *Journal of Allied Health, 39*(4), 280–286.

Flannery, J. (1993). Psychometric properties of a cognitive functional scale for patients with traumatic brain injury. *Western Journal of Nursing Research, 15*(4), 465–482.

Ginsberg, S. M., Friberg, J. C., & Visconti, C. F. (2016). Diagnostic reasoning by experienced speech-language pathologists and student clinicians. *Contemporary Issues in Communication Science and Disorders, 43,* 87–97.

Goldman, R. & Fristoe, M. (2015). *Goldman-Fristoe Test of Articulation 3 (GFTA-3).* Pearson.

Gonzalez, L., Nielsen, A., & Lasater, K. (2021). Developing students' clinical reasoning skills: A faculty guide. *The Journal of Nursing Education, 60*(9), 485–493. https://doi.org /10.3928/01484834-20210708-01

Halls, D., Murray, C., & Sellar, B. (2021). Why allied health professionals use evidence-based clinical guidelines in stroke rehabilitation: A systematic review and meta-synthesis of qualitative studies. *Clinical Rehabilitation, 35*(11), 1611–1626. https://doi.org/10.1177/02692155211012324

Helm-Estabrooks, N. (2001). *Cognitive Linguistic Quick Test.* Pearson.

Hersh, D., Worrall, L., Howe, T., Sherratt, S., & Davidson, B. (2012). *SMARTER* goal setting in aphasia rehabilitation. *Aphasiology, 26*(2), 220–233. https://doi.org/10.1080/0268 7038.2011.640392

Huhn, K., Black, L., Jensen, G. M., & Deutsch, J. E. (2011). Construct validity of the health science reasoning test. *Journal of Allied Health, 40*(4), 181–186.

Ilgen, J. S., Eva, K. W., & Regehr, G. (2016). What's in a label? Is diagnosis the start or the end of clinical reasoning? *Journal of General Internal Medicine, 31*(4), 435–437. https://doi.org/10.1007/s11606-016-3592-7

Individuals with Disabilities Education Act. (2004). *Section 1400.* https://sites.ed.gov/idea/statute-chapter-33/subchapter-i/1400

Kagan, A., Simmons-Mackie, N., Victor, J. C., Carline-Rowland, A., Hoch, J., Huijbregts, M., . . . Mok, A. (2013). *Assessment for Living with Aphasia, Second Edition (ALA).* Aphasia Institute.

Kaplan, E., Goodglass, H., Weintraub, S., & Segal, O. (2001). *Boston Naming Test.* Pro-Ed.

Katz, J. D., & George, D. T. (2019). Reclaiming magical incantation in graduate medical education. *Clinical Rheumatology, 39*(3), 703–707. https://doi.org/10.1007/s10067-019-04812-x

Khan M. L., & Lewis P. N. (2015). *Khan-Lewis Phonological Analysis, Third Edition.* Pearson.

Kleim, J.A., & Jones, T.A. (2008). Principles of experience-dependent neural plasticity: Implications for rehabilitation after brain damage. *Journal of Speech, Language, and Hearing Research, 51*(1): S225–239. https://doi.org/10.1044/1092-4388(2008/018)

Macdonald, S. (2005) *Functional Assessment of Verbal Reasoning and Executive Strategies. (FAVRES).* CCD Publishing.

Marian, V., Blumenfeld, H. K., & Kaushanskaya, M. (2007). The Language Experience and Proficiency Questionnaire (LEAP-Q): Assessing language profiles in bilinguals and multilinguals. *Journal of Speech, Language, and Hearing Research, 50*(4), 940–967. https://doi.org/10.1044/1092-4388(2007/067)

Moore, R. (2018). Beyond 80-percent accuracy: Consider alternative objective criteria in writing your treatment goals. *The ASHA Leader, 23*(5).

Nawka, T., Verdonck-de Leeuw, I. M., De Bodt, M., Guimaraes, I., Holmberg, E. B., Rosen, C. . . . Konerding, U. (2009).

Item reduction of the Voice Handicap Index based on the original version and on European translations. *Folia Phoniatrica et Logopaedica, 61*(1), 37–48. https://doi.org/10.1159/000200767

Nobriga, C., & St. Clair, J. (2018). Training goal writing: A practical and systematic approach. *Perspectives of the ASHA Special Interest Groups, 3,*11 36–47. https://doi.org/10.1044/persp3.SIG11.36

Paradis, J., Emmerzael, K., & Duncan, T. S. (2010). Assessment of English language learners: Using parent report on first language development. *Journal of Communication Disorders, 43*(6), 474–497. https://doi.org/10.1016/j.jcomdis.2010.01.002

Paradis, M., & Libben, G. (1987). *The assessment of bilingual aphasia.* Psychology Press. https://www.mcgill.ca/linguistics/research/bat

Peña, E. D., Gutiérrez-Clellen, V. F., Iglesias, A., Goldstein, B., & Bedore, L. M. (2018). *Bilingual English Spanish Assessment (BESA).* Brookes.

Poventud, L. S., Corbett, N. L., Daunic, A. P., Aydin, B., Lane, H., & Smith, S. W. (2015). Developing social-emotional vocabulary to support self-regulation for young children at risk for emotional and behavioral problems. *International Journal of School and Cognitive Psychology, 2*(143), 2.

Rencic, J. (2011). Twelve tips for teaching expertise in clinical reasoning. *Medical Teacher, 33*(11), 887–892. https://doi.org/10.3109/0142159x.2011.558142

Richards, J. B., Hayes, M. M., & Schwartzstein, R. M. (2020). Teaching clinical reasoning and critical thinking: From cognitive theory to practical application. *Chest, 158*(4), 1617–1628. https://doi.org/10.1016/j.chest.2020.05.525

Riley, G., & Bakker, K. (2009). *SSI-4: Stuttering Severity Instrument.* Pro-Ed.

Schuwirth, L. W., Durning, S. J., & King, S. M. (2020). Assessment of clinical reasoning: Three evolutions of thought. *Diagnosis, 7*(3), 191–196. https://doi.org/10.1515/dx-2019-0096

Shin, H. S. (2019). Reasoning processes in clinical reasoning: From the perspective of cognitive psychology. *Korean Journal of Medical Education, 31*(4), 299–308. https://doi.org/10.3946/kjme.2019.140

Simmons-Mackie, N., Kagan, A., Victor, J. C., Carling-Rowland, A., Mok, A., Hoch, J. S., . . . Streiner, D. L. (2014). The Assessment for Living with Aphasia: Reliability and construct validity. *International Journal of Speech-Language Pathology, 16*(1), 82–94.

Tesoro, M. G. (2012). Effects of using the developing nurses' thinking model on nursing students' diagnostic accuracy. *Journal of Nursing Education, 51*(8), 436–443. https://doi.org/10.3928/01484834-20120615-01

Thampy, H., Willert, E., & Ramani, S. (2019). Assessing clinical reasoning: Targeting the higher levels of the pyramid. *Journal of General Internal Medicine, 34*(8), 1631–1636. https://doi.org/10.1007/s11606-019-04953-4

Torres, I. G. (2013). Write targeted treatment goals: Use these tricks to set goals that your client can hit and that you can measure. *The ASHA Leader, 18*(11).

Wainwright, S. F., & McGinnis, P. Q. (2009). Factors that influence the clinical decision-making of rehabilitation professionals in long-term care settings. *Journal of Allied Health, 38*(3), 143–151.

Wiederholt L. J., & Bryant, R. B. (2012). *Gray Oral Reading Fifth Edition (GORT-5)*. Pearson.

Wigg, H. E., Secord A. W., & Semel, E. (2020) *Clinical Evaluation of Language Fundamentals Preschool-3 Screening Test*. Pearson.

World Health Organization. (n.d.). *International Classification of Functioning, Disability and Health (ICF)*. World Health

Organization. https://www.who.int/standards/classifications/international-classification-of-functioning-disability-and-health

Yaruss, J. S., & Quesal, R. W. (2016). *Overall Assessment of the Speaker's Experience of Stuttering-Teen (OASES-T)*. Stuttering Therapy Resources.

Yorkston, K., Beukelman, D. R., & Tice, R. (1996). *Sentence Intelligibility Test [Measurement instrument]*. Tice Technologies.

Young, M. E., Thomas, A., Lubarsky, S., Gordon, D., Gruppen, L. D., Rencic, J., . . . Durning, S. J. (2020). Mapping clinical reasoning literature across the health professions: A scoping review. *BMC Medical Education, 20*(1), 1–11.

Zimmerman, L. I., Steiner, G. V., & Pond, E. R. (2011). *Preschool Language Scales, Fifth Edition*. Pearson.

Index

Note: Page numbers in **bold** reference non-text material.